HEALTHY

MADE EASY

A HOW-TO GUIDE ON SUSTAINING HEALTHIER EATING HABITS

BY MITCHELL THOMPSON

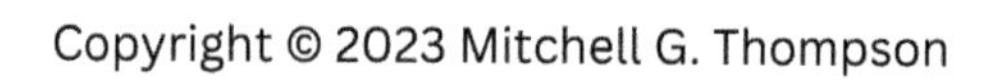

Copyright © 2023 Mitchell G. Thompson

All rights reserved. No part(s) of this book may be reproduced, distributed, or transmitted in any form, or by any means, or stored in a database or retrieval systems without prior expressed written permission of the author of this book

ISBN: 979-8-218-30912-1

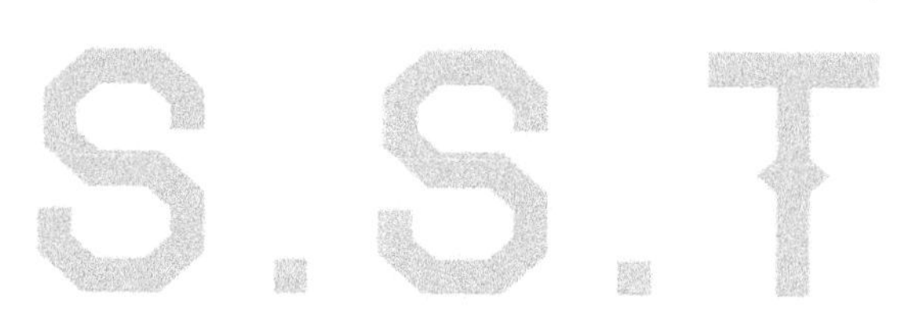

Table of Contents

Chapter 1

The Importance of Healthy Living

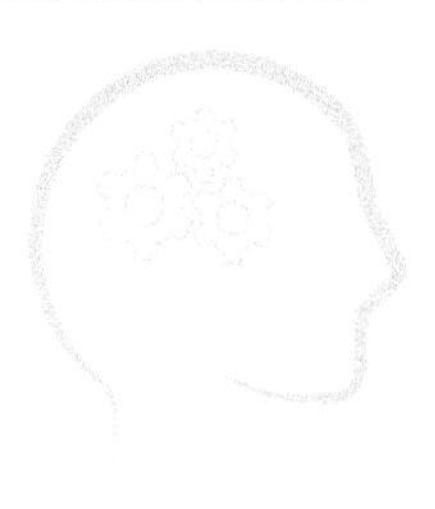

Do you want to feel like your best self?

Do you want to be more energized and have a better sense of fulfillment?

Do you want to know how to improve your life and well-being?

I had to answer these questions when I was at my worst, and I continue to fulfill the response of "yes" in order to sustain myself at my best.

The problem with becoming your best self in the 21st century is the weighted blanket of comfort that modern society provides. We're fortunate to have the luxuries of air conditioning, easily accessible running water, efficient transportation, and round-the-clock access to food. In many ways, modern life pampers us with its conveniences.

And being your best self isn't convenient. You have to earn it.

In fact, living a happy, healthy, and more fulfilling life is less convenient than living a less happy, unhealthy, and less fulfilling life.

Conveniency may make you happy now, but it is not a sustainable happiness. The whisper of convenience is both a comforting lullaby and a stealthy saboteur.

It's a peculiar aspect of human nature that, while we often seek the path of least resistance, we also yearn for meaningful growth and fulfillment. It's as if we stand at the crossroads of convenience and aspiration, grappling with the tension between immediate gratification and long-term reward.

Convenience, with its seductive temptation, often appears as the easier road to travel. It promises quick fixes, instant pleasures, and the comfort of familiarity. Much like a well-trodden path, it requires minimal effort, inviting us to follow along without questioning where it leads.

Dripping water hollows stone through persistence.

Picture bad habits as a dripping faucet, each droplet representing a small, seemingly harmless convenience in your daily routine. If we put a rock underneath the dripping faucet, at first there would be no immediate effects. And just like raindrops on a rock, one alone won't create much of an impact. So it's easy to justify convenient choices, believing that they won't significantly alter the shape of your life. However, if those droplets persist over time, they will surely erode the rock's surface. Remember, *it's the persistence of convenient choices that can slowly erode your well-being*, leaving you dissatisfied with a future that you have crafted yourself.

On the flip side, the journey of growth and creation demands something more profound—effort, resilience, and the willingness to embrace the unknown. It's like forging a new trail through uncharted terrain. And being your healthiest self, at this point in your life, is likely uncharted terrain. This path, though inherently more challenging, holds the promise of something far greater. It offers the opportunity to consciously shape your own life and cultivate a rich future full of intention and consideration.

Here's the catch though: while it's relatively easy to drift down the river of convenience and relinquish control to your current habits of instant gratification, the act of purposefully steering toward the path of growth requires sustained deliberate effort. It's akin to fighting a conveniency current and thus swimming upstream. This demands that we fight against the tide of convenience and consciously choose the more uncomfortable route.

Is it convenient to help an old lady cross the street when you're heading in the opposite direction? No, but the subtlety of the inconvenience pales in comparison to the minimal effort it would take to help an old lady cross the street.

Is it convenient to protect a random child who ran up to you and is getting chased by a dog? No, but if you wouldn't help an innocent child who is getting chased by a dog, then eating better is the least of your concerns.

Over time, the conveniency of your bad habits will catch up with you and your future self will ultimately be unhappy. Conveniency won't fulfill you the same way earning things will - especially with regard to your health. It's sad because the conveniency of modern life nearly forces us to choose the less healthy and less fulfilled path for ourselves.

"Why would I go hunt for my food when I can buy hunks of food at the store?"

"Why would I go buy all of the ingredients to make a cheeseburger and fries (and then spend the time cooking the meal, then subsequently cleaning after the meal) when I can go get the food in a faster way?"

"Why would I exercise and be fit when there's nothing to run from, fight against, or hunt down?"

"Why endure the harder thing when the easier option is right there, conveniently in front of me?

In this paradox, we find the heart of the matter: it's often simpler to let conveniency guide us down a path of gradual erosion, where our habits and choices gradually reshape our life's path, sometimes in ways we never intended. The erosion happens so subtly that it can catch us off guard, leaving us dissatisfied with a future that we've unwittingly shaped. Whereas creating and nurturing positive habits, like tending to ourself as if we were a flourishing garden, necessitates patience and persistence.

It requires us to recognize the scent of instant gratification and consciously opt for the long-term reward. In this journey, we step into the role of creators, architects of our own life, deliberately sculpting the future we desire. But that starts with setting and achieving goals - which isn't convenient. Setting and achieving goals, no matter how big or small, is crucial for a more fulfilling life.

The key to being healthy and living longer is simple: *improve circulation and decrease inflammation.* As a seasoned, hands-on personal trainer, I can attest to the straightforward nature of achieving these goals: improve your diet to decrease inflammation and enhance your movement to increase circulation.

Circulation is simply the body's ability to thoroughly transport essential biochemicals (blood, nutrients, oxygen, hormones, etc.) through the blood and dispense them appropriately throughout the entire body, which is hindered by chronic inflammation. Mastering our movement, or biomechanics (meaning how we stand, walk, and move in space), primarily remedies our poor circulation. However, when it comes to reducing inflammation, the food we eat becomes the ultimate determining factor. Inflammation, at its core, is the body's response to injury or infection. So it's a necessary process that helps us heal. Yet, in today's world, excessive inflammation plagues us and has become the primary contributor to many chronic diseases.

Our gut, often referred to as our 'second brain,' plays a vital role in managing inflammation. A healthy gut lining is crucial because it acts as a barrier, preventing harmful substances from leaking into our bloodstream to trigger systemic inflammation. To put it into perspective, envision your digestive system as a plumbing network: your mouth serves as your home's toilet, while your anus acts as the city's sewage system.

Just as you'd only flush materials down your home's toilet that won't obstruct the plumbing or harm its pipe-lining, your gut must maintain the integrity of its plumbing to prevent chronic inflammation. Ultimately, a compromised gut health compromises the entire body.

When this lining is compromised, as it often is due to poor dietary choices, it can lead to increased gut permeability (meaning how easily things can pass through the gut barrier). This condition is referred to as 'leaky gut syndrome,' and it results in toxins and undigested food particles breaching into the body and setting off a cascade of inflammation. It's similar to a compromised lining within the plumbing system of your home, and how sewage would begin to seep into the foundation of your house. Except your house is your body, and the effects of seeping sewage causes a chronic inflammatory response. Like a slow-burning fire within us, a compromised gut lining raises the risk of developing chronic diseases such as heart disease, diabetes, autoimmune disorders, and even mental health issues. All of these issues stem from an overactive immune system diligently responding to the consequences of poor dietary choices. This is a form of metabolic dysfunction, and having metabolic dysfunction is also known as being *metabolically unhealthy.*

And the sad reality is that over 90% of Americans are metabolically unhealthy, which means only 10% of us (or less) are eating as healthy as we should.[1] As we dig deeper, we'll uncover the harsh truth that poor dietary habits are at the root of chronic inflammation plaguing our bodies.

This implies that a significant portion of Americans are currently dealing with chronic inflammation, often unknowingly, and particularly within the gut. The path to living healthier and longer begins with nurturing our gut health. A diet rich in nutrients that include anti-inflammatory foods, soluble fiber-rich vegetables, and overall clean-sourced produce will be the secret formula to being your healthiest self. Combine this with mindful movement and we're on the right track to reducing inflammation, improving circulation, and safeguarding our long-term health.

Eating healthy is not about deprivation. It's about making sustainable choices that will nourish your body and mind. I always tell my clients that a healthy diet deserves dessert every night. Think of healthy eating as a percentage distribution, aiming for a minimum of 80% clean eating and allowing for 20% flexibility for indulgence. When you consistently prioritize clean eating, you 'earn the right' to enjoy occasional rewards within that 20%. Now, qualifying that reward and ensuring it does not exceed that 20% is a separate conversation altogether.

The ultimate goal is to establish a sustainable ratio that aligns with a healthy lifestyle, never falling below the 80% clean and 20% indulgence guideline. By providing these rewards and finding the right balance, my clients are motivated to make positive choices and cultivate sustainable habits for long-term success.

As hinted at earlier, imagine a slow burning fire (like an unsupervised bonfire) that continues to burn when, at some point, it needs to be extinguished or it could turn into a wildfire. Similarly, when we subject our tissues (particularly our organs and intestines) to chronic and excessive inflammation, it leads to damage and counteracts the healing process.

Moreover, an overactive immune system due to persistent inflammation can create a *tolerance to the autoimmune response* - diminishing its overall effectiveness. This means that our immune system becomes desensitized, which impacts its ability to function optimally in other areas of the body. This results in you getting sick easier, getting injured easier, and generally increasing your susceptibility to discomfort, disease, and eventually death.

Another important aspect to consider is the role of movement and biomechanics. Because we sit so much in modern times, it has deformed our natural anatomy, specifically in regard to how we stand and walk. To put it in perspective, our anatomy is designed to walk an upwards of 15,000 steps per day, whereas the average modern American walks around 3,000 steps per day.

Poor movement patterns and biomechanical issues simply exacerbates our poor health. When our joints are compressed, and our muscles and connective tissues remain tight due to gnarled imbalances, it further fuels the flames of inflammation. It's similar to adding more fuel to the already burning fire that needs to be extinguished. Consequently, this combination of poor movement and an overly active immune system is what accelerates degeneration and leads to a multitude of health complications.

To protect our well-being, it's essential to take a comprehensive approach that addresses inflammation, movement, and immune system function. Employing healthier movement patterns (correcting biomechanical issues) and making mindful dietary choices allows us to reduce excessive inflammation, improve our body's circulation, and foster long-term sustainable healthy habits.

This book is a comprehensive view at the dietary side of things.

So how do you eat healthy?

It's really not that hard, but it does require an understanding of the biological variance that exists among every individual when it comes to dietary preferences, needs, and responses. Simply put: everyone is different, and *there is no one-size-fits-all approach to what constitutes "healthy eating."* Like most things, a lack of understanding or a lack of knowledge will likely result in failure. And if you've failed at trying to eat healthy before, it's likely due to your lack of knowledge on how to actually eat healthy; taking into account your lifestyle, your unique genetic makeup, and your body's responses to certain foods.

And that's okay. That is what this entire book is for: to equip you with the knowledge to start making healthier choices in your day-to-day eating, while recognizing that *there is no one-size-fits-all approach to nutrition.* Start by incorporating small, manageable changes to your diet, as we will explore in the following sections.

And don't forget to enjoy your food! Eating healthy doesn't mean you have to give up your favorite foods. Just make sure you're enjoying them in moderation, while being mindful of how your body responds. For all you know, some of your favorite foods are yet to be discovered, as many healthy foods can taste better (and will taste better, over time) than heavily processed foods. It's a sustainable journey, not a final destination, and it takes time and effort to make healthy eating a habit. But it's worth it, and your future self will thank you every day for the rest of your life for simply starting today with a better understanding of your unique nutritional needs.

When you are nourishing your body with nutritious foods, you can feel your best, live your best, reduce the risk of chronic diseases, and embrace a longer, healthier, happier, and more prosperous life.

Eating better not only impacts your physical health but also has a profound effect on your mental and emotional health. A cleaner diet provides essential nutrients that support the production of improved hormones and neural chemicals, specifically serotonin, to enhance mood and defog your mind. Furthermore, it empowers you to cultivate stronger connections in your relationships - but more importantly your relationship with yourself. With increased energy, mental clarity, and emotional stability, you'll become a better version of you in all facets of your life. And a better you is a better friend to your friends, a better partner to your partner, and a better relative to your loved ones. Remember, embracing healthy eating is a continual journey, and this book serves as your guide to making informed choices and developing sustainable eating habits.

Start with small changes, enjoy the process, and celebrate every step forward. Your future self will be grateful for the positive steps you take today towards a healthier and more fulfilling tomorrow.

Chapter 2

Understanding Nutrition Basics

In this chapter, we will lay the foundation of your nutritional knowledge by exploring the basics of nutrition. Understanding the role of macronutrients and micronutrients, the principles of a balanced diet, and the importance of portion control will empower you to make informed choices about the foods you consume.

Macronutrients and Micronutrients:

Macro = big, micro = small.

To fuel our bodies and support optimal functioning, we require macronutrients and micronutrients. Though micronutrients (vitamins and minerals) are essential, the main thing the average person should worry about is their macronutrients.

Simply worry about the big nutrients.

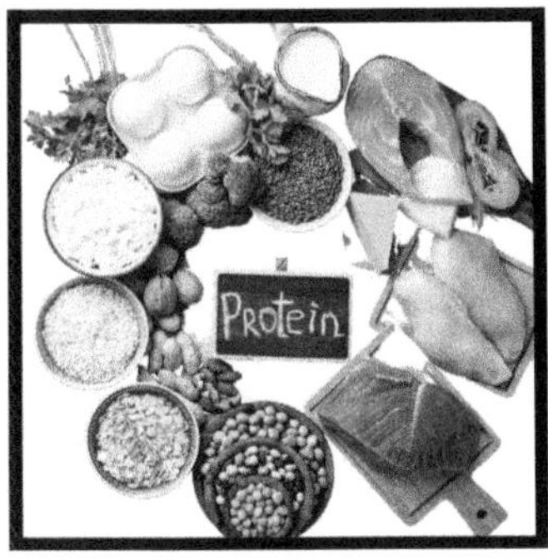

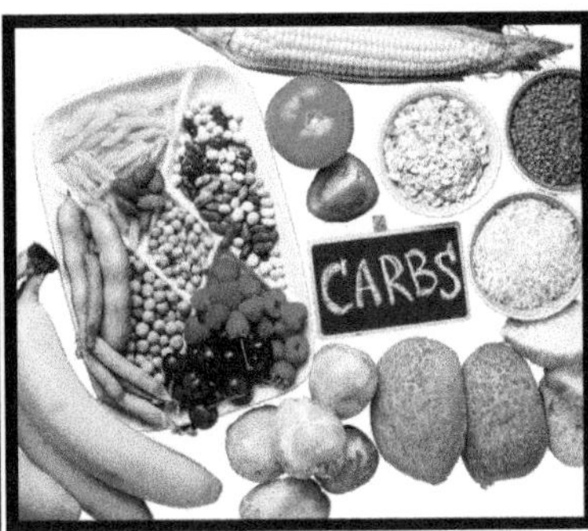

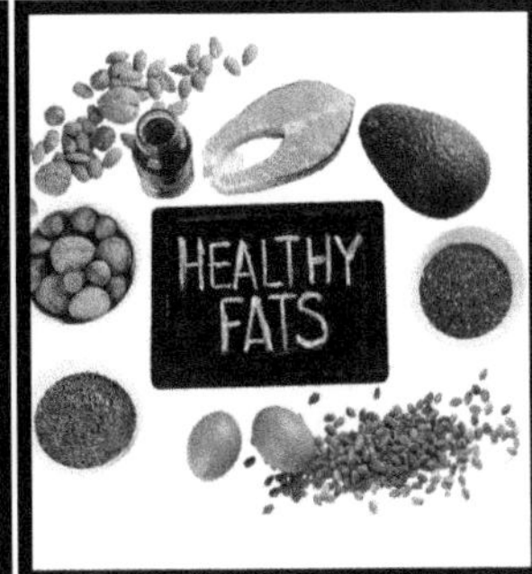

Our macronutrients are carbohydrates, fats and proteins. While calories aren't a nutrient, since they are technically a measure of energy like volts or watts, we will consider them as an important variable to measure in our diet. These variables can be compared to the elements of nature, where each element plays a crucial role in our bodies functioning harmoniously.

When macronutrients are digested and metabolized by the body, they are broken down into simpler forms that can be used for energy production. This energy is measured in calories. Each gram of carbohydrate and protein provides 4 calories, while each gram of fat provides 9 calories (don't worry, you won't have to remember stuff like this). The body requires calories from these macronutrients for a multitude of physiological functions such as building and repairing tissues, supporting the immune system, and regulating various biological processes.

Calories

Calories represent the energy we derive from food. Calories are important with regard to gaining and losing weight. Since we're all different, we all burn calories at different rates depending on our genetics, job, and general way of being. This "base rate of calorie burning" (meaning the amount of calories we burn for just being) for each individual is known as a 'basal metabolic rate' and the average basal metabolic rate (BMR) for men is between 1600-1800 calories and for women it is between 1400-1600 calories.[1] This 'BMR' only includes the calories burned from your body being at rest - this does not account for any calories burned from working out. From my experience, calories are less important to focus on rather than protein, carbs, and fats because prioritizing the macronutrient numbers generally equates to an adequate caloric count as well as insuring you are not malnourished.

However, it is important to note your BMR and cross reference it with how many calories you intake. **If you want to lose weight, you should eat less calories than you burn.** So if your BMR is 1700 calories per day and you burn an extra 300 calories from a workout, then you should eat less than 2000 calories in order to lose weight. If you want to gain weight, then the process is an inverse function, meaning you would eat more than your BMR + the calories burned from a workout. If you do not workout, then you will need to eat less than your BMR - even though it is crucial that you get some form of caloric burn from physical activity regularly. If you do not workout, then it will be a lot harder to lose weight in general (because working out increases circulation...a key component to becoming your healthiest self) and therefore you will yield less results from the healthier eating altogether.

And working out does not have to be an arduous chore...it's a lot easier than you think! All you have to do is fix your posture and fix the way you walk, but that is a conversation for another book altogether.

Carbohydrates

Carbs fuel our muscles, brain, and other vital organs. Carbohydrates come in two forms: simple and complex. Simple carbs, found in foods like packaged snacks, candy, and refined sugars, provide quick energy bursts. Complex carbs, found in starches, fruits, and vegetables, provide sustained energy and essential nutrients. Whether a carb is simple or complex determines its glycemic index (GI), which measures how quickly a carbohydrate gets digested and raises blood sugar levels. The term 'glycemic' refers to the carbohydrate's glucose density, as all carbs are eventually broken down into glucose, a type of sugar.

Foods with a high glycemic index (typically simple carbs, like table sugar/candy) cause a rapid increase in blood sugar levels because they are dense with immediate glucose. In contrast, those with a low glycemic index (usually complex carbs, like fruits and veggies) have a more gradual, slow-digestive impact. However, it's essential to note that not all simple carbs are high GI, and not all complex carbs are low GI. Factors like fiber content and food processing can influence a food's GI. To get a more accurate picture of how a food affects blood sugar, we consider the glycemic load (GL), which factors in both the GI and the portion size of the food. Lower GL foods are generally better for maintaining stable blood sugar levels.

As Americans, we should focus on foods with lower glycemic loads, opt for minimally processed options, and balance them with other nutrient-rich foods. Remember that while the glycemic index is important, it's the overall glycemic load that truly matters, and this can be easily managed by being mindful of portion sizes.

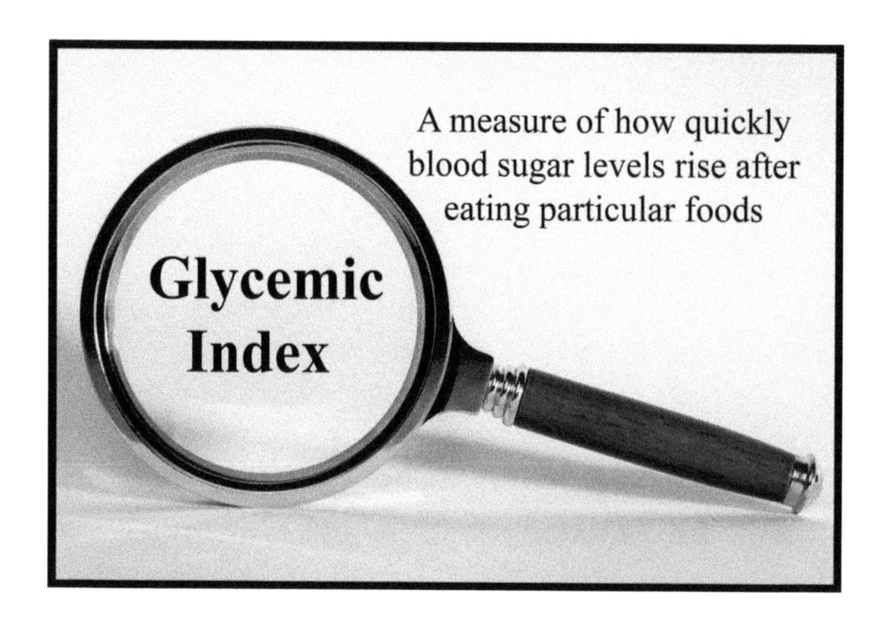

Glycemic Index Food Examples

Low Glycemic Index (GI) Foods:

(SST Approved)

1. Apples
2. Cherries
3. Lentils
4. Greek yogurt
5. Walnuts
6. Avocado
7. Berries (e.g., strawberries, blueberries)
8. Non-starchy vegetables (e.g., broccoli, cauliflower)
9. Non-cow Dairy

(NOT SST Approved, for now)

1. Cow Dairy
2. Raw carrots
3. Hummus
4. Kidney beans
5. All-Bran cereal
6. Green peas
7. Peanuts
8. Cashews
9. Soy milk
10. Green beans

Medium Glycemic Index (GI) Foods:

(SST Approved)

1. Sweet potatoes
2. Pineapple
3. Peaches
4. Kiwi
5. Grapes
6. Banana
7. Beets
8. Sweetened yogurt
9. Plantains
10. Cantaloup

(NOT SST Approved, for now)

1. Bulgur (cracked wheat)
2. Whole grain spaghetti
3. Barley
4. Rye bread
5. Brown rice
6. Oat bran
7. Basmati rice
8. Pita bread (whole wheat)
9. Buckwheat

High Glycemic Index (GI) Foods:

(SST Approved)

1. White Rice
2. White Bread
3. Pineapple juice
4. Dates
5. Rice cakes
6. Popcorn (popped)
7. Pretzels
8. Mashed potatoes
9. Beets
10. Watermelon

(NOT SST Approved, for now)

1. Instant rice
2. Rice cakes (whole grain)
3. Bagels (whole wheat)
4. Granola
5. Millet
6. Short-grain white rice
7. Pumpkin seeds

Dietary Fats

Dietary fats, which are also known as lipids or triglycerides, primarily serve as stored sources of energy in our bodies. ***Dietary fats do not make you fat.*** In fact, ***excess calorie intake (namely from carbs) is what makes you fat.*** When you eat excessive carbs, your body will convert it into *body fat* to store in the form of triglycerides.

Triglycerides act as energy reserves, providing a concentrated form of fuel that can be utilized when needed. Our body prefers to use glucose, but will store triglycerides and use it as energy when glucose is unavailable. Again, when we eat in excess, specifically when we eat too many carbs, the gluttenous glucose gets converted into triglycerides and is stored as "body fat" or adipose tissue, which is how and why we "get fat."

There are two main types of dietary fats: saturated and unsaturated. Saturated fats are found in animal products like meat, dairy, and eggs. They are also found in a few plant oils, like coconut oil and palm oil. Unsaturated fats are found in plant-based foods like nuts, seeds, and avocados. They are also found in most oils, like olive oil and canola oil. Fatty acids from both are essential components of our diet and play a crucial role in our health. They also interact with cholesterol, another important substance in our bodies. Cholesterol, a fat-like substance, is produced naturally by our liver and obtained through certain foods. When it comes to cholesterol, there are two types that are often mentioned: HDL (high-density lipoprotein) and LDL (low-density lipoprotein). HDL cholesterol is often referred to as "good" cholesterol because it helps remove LDL cholesterol from the bloodstream and transports it to the liver for processing and elimination.

Low HDL numbers are associated with increased cardiovascular disease, and is the underlying cause of metabolic dysfunction.[2] Certain types of fatty acids can affect the levels of HDL and LDL cholesterol in the body. For example, unsaturated fats are considered to be healthier than saturated fats because they can help raise 'good' cholesterol (HDL) levels and protect against heart disease.

It's important to strike a balance in our fat intake by opting for healthier sourced fats while moderating the intake of poorly sourced fats. This is best exemplified through grass-fed meat and dairy being a better source of saturated fat than grain-fed meat and dairy. Or the unsaturated fats from olive oil being healthier than the unsaturated fats from industrialized seed oils.

Protein

Protein is essential for the structure, function, growth, and repair of tissues in our bodies. They are made up of amino acids, which act as the building blocks for tissues, enzymes, hormones, and antibodies. Protein is critical for the growth, development, and maintenance of muscle mass, as well as general health and immune function. Protein-rich foods play a crucial role in regulating hunger and reducing cravings. Protein takes longer to digest, keeping us feeling fuller for an extended time while stabilizing our blood sugar levels and curbing the desire for sugary and unhealthy foods.

Most Americans are protein deficient, meaning they are not getting nearly enough protein on a daily basis. Not only will increasing your protein intake curve cravings and make you feel more full, but it will also allow you to meet your daily recommended intake for protein in order to maintain optimal health standards. I advise my female clients to consume *at least* 80 grams of protein per day and my male clients to consume *at least* 120 grams of protein per day. Ultimately, your protein intake depends on your activity level and your goals for muscle growth.

Technically, from a clinical standpoint, the recommended daily average of protein you should consume is only .36 grams per pound of body weight.[3] However, depending on your level of physical activity, your body will need more protein. The amount of protein you should aim for depends on the intensity of your fitness regimen. For individuals with more rigorous fitness protocols, I suggest increasing protein intake to meet the demands of muscle recovery and support enhanced protein synthesis. For more intense fitness regimens, I would recommend .8 to 1.2 grams of protein per pound of body weight.

Just as the four elements of nature interact and contribute to the equilibrium of the world, carbohydrates, fats, protein, and calories interact within our bodies to maintain optimal health and function. It's essential to understand the role of each element and consume them in appropriate quantities as part of a well-rounded diet.

And this is how I have helped countless clients (both in person and virtually) through simply tracking and knowing their daily macronutrient intake. Meaning, if you can learn how to set a goal of x number of protein, carbs, fats, and calories per day and can subsequently meet those macronutrient goals daily, then you will be **guaranteed** success in becoming healthier.

Micronutrients, such as vitamins and minerals, are needed in smaller quantities but are equally important for various bodily functions, including immune support, bone health, and cell regulation. And as a seasoned health professional, I can assure you that if you simply worry about macronutrient maintenance, then you will achieve an adequate amount of micronutrient nourishment that will not require for you to track/measure/qualify your micronutrient intake. So long your food is predominantly organic and well sourced, your micronutrient standards should be met. Once you've established a healthy enough diet, you will only "need" to take a few supplements for the sake of optimization. Supplements like *vitamin D+K*, *magnesium glycinate*, *methylated vitamin B9 (5-MTHF)*, and *omega-3s* will be staples even if you eat optimally.

In the next few pages, I will show you how to properly track your macronutrients and what exactly that looks like. Once you've tracked your macronutrients for a few weeks, you'll start building a habit of recognizing measurement sizes, the nutrient density of foods, and how much you should or shouldn't eat. At first, you might find it challenging to gauge the exact portion size of a cup of rice or the weight of a cut of meat. However, with consistent measuring and diligent tracking, you'll soon develop the skill to estimate your macros without needing to track your food.

How to track your food

Tracking your food isn't that hard, it just takes some learning. And once you've learned, it then just takes practice.

1. Google "Macro Calculator" (I've always used calculator.net, but they all essentially do the same thing)

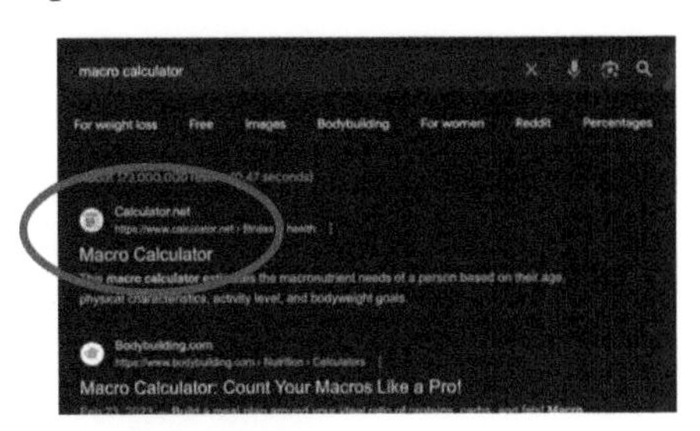

2. Fill out the appropriate information as best as you can

(Be more conservative in your answers here)

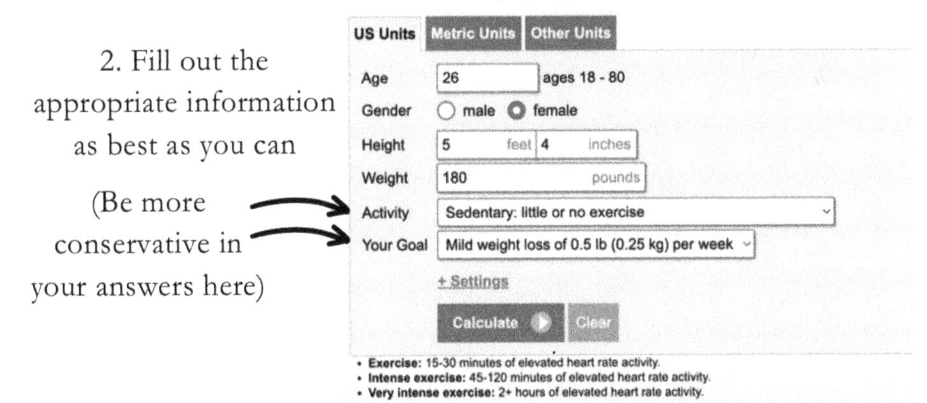

3. Make sure to check the "High Protein" option

4. Try to eat the recommended daily intake of each macronutrient. Give yourself the freedom to be off a little bit, but try to stay within a (+/-) 10g to 20g window and (+/-) 100 calories. This means try not to eat more or less than 10-20g outside of your macronutrient goal, and keep your calories within 100 calories of your caloric goal.

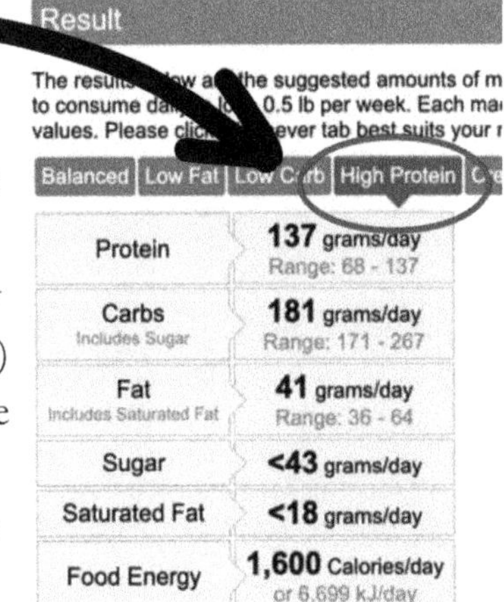

Macronutrient Tracking Example:

Once you've got your macronutrient numbers, it's all about learning how to measure your food and keeping track of your daily nutrient intake.

Thank goodness we've got technology, because tracking your macros the old-fashion way is painstakingly tedious. Nowadays, there are thousands of apps that will help you track your macro and micronutrients. Again, for now, simply worry about your macro nutrients.

Depending on which app you use will qualify how you actually track your food. I use MyFitnessPal, but many of my clients find other apps that they like better. Just like the macro-calculator choice, the food-tracking choice doesn't make much of a difference.

Most of the food-tracking apps have some form of a "Diary" or "Food Log" where you can actually look up the foods you are eating and see their nutritional values. To make things even more convenient, **most of these apps have nearly every/any food item in a typical grocery store** and their exact nutritional makeup.

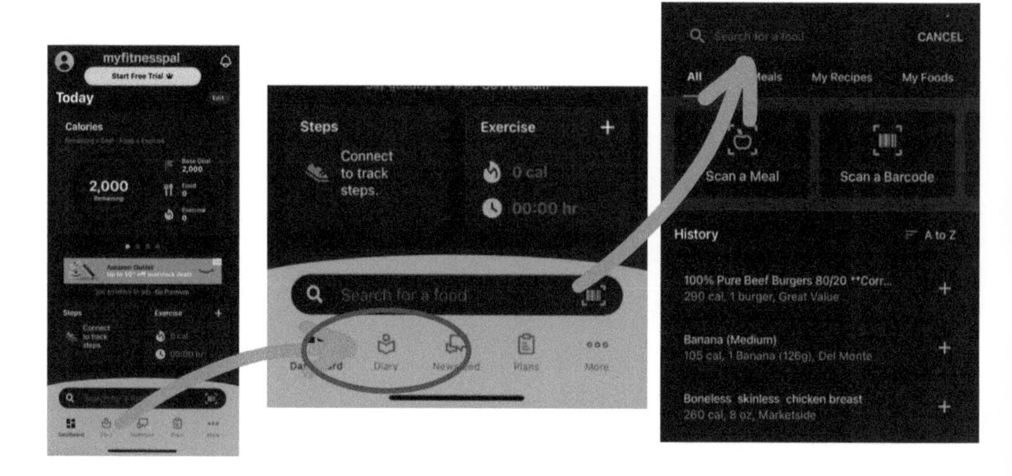

MEASURING YOUR FOOD

- **Gather Your Tools: Log everything you eat and drink! To start measuring your food, you'll need some basic tools:**
  - Kitchen scale: A digital kitchen scale is a must. It provides precise measurements in grams or ounces.
  - Measuring cups and spoons: These are handy for measuring liquids, grains, and smaller portions.
  - Food diary or mobile app: To record what you eat, you can use a notebook or a food tracking app on your smartphone.

- **Weigh Solid Foods:**

a. Place your empty plate or bowl on the kitchen scale.
b. Turn on the scale and set it to zero (tare) with the empty plate.
c. Add your food to the plate.
d. Read the weight displayed on the scale in grams or ounces.
e. Record the weight in your food diary or app.

- **Measure Liquids:**

a. Use a liquid measuring cup for liquids.
b. Fill the measuring cup to the desired level and read the measurement.
c. Record the measurement in your food diary or app.

- **Portion Control:**

a. Use measuring cups and spoons for foods like rice, pasta, or cereal.
b. Fill the measuring cup or spoon, leveling it off for accuracy.
c. Record the portion size.

- **Practice Estimation:**

a. When eating out or in situations where you can't measure precisely, try to estimate portion sizes.
b. With time, you'll get better at estimating.

- **Be Consistent:**

a. Try to measure and track your food consistently.
b. Over time, this will help you understand your eating habits and make healthier choices.

- **Monitor Your Progress:**

a. Regularly review your food diary or app to track your eating patterns.
b. Make adjustments based on your goals, whether it's weight loss, maintenance, or better nutrition.

- **Seek Guidance:**

If you have specific dietary goals or medical conditions, consult with a healthcare professional or nutritionist for personalized guidance.

Let's use an example from one of my client's typical days.

John Doe's Macronutrient breakdown:

2,100 calories/day
160g protein/day
190g carbs/day
80g fat/day

Adjust portion sizes to your macros. Remember, it's always okay to be under on carbs and fat!

John Doe has to eat ***at least 150g of protein*, *no more than 200g carbs*, *no more than 90g of fat***, and ***no more than 2,200 calories***.

Breakfast [8am]

Approx. 350 calories
Protein: 20g
Fat: 26g
Carbs: 11g

- Scrambled Eggs (3 large eggs): 210 calories, 18g protein, 15g fat, 0g carbs
- Avocado (1/2 avocado): 120 calories, 2g protein, 11g fat, 6g carbs
- Fresh Blueberries (1/2 cup): 20 calories, 0g protein, 0g fat, 5g carbs

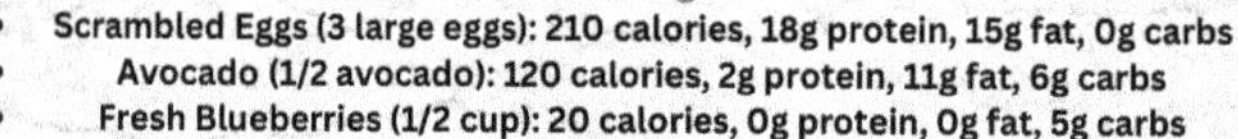

Morning Snack [10am]

Approx. 200 calories
Protein: 17g
Fat: 4g
Carbs: 8g

- Greek Yogurt (6 oz): 150 calories, 15g protein, 0g fat, 6g carbs
- Almonds (1 oz, about 23 almonds): 50 calories, 2g protein, 4g fat, 2g carbs

Lunch [noon]

Approx. 486 calories
Protein: 60g
Fat: 18g
Carbs: 20g

- Grilled Chicken Breast (6 oz): 270 calories, 54g protein, 4g fat, 0g carbs
- Roasted Brussels Sprouts (1 cup): 66 calories, 3g protein, 0g fat, 13g carbs
- Sautéed Zucchini (1 cup): 30 calories, 2g protein, 0g fat, 6g carbs
- Avocado Oil (1 tablespoon for cooking): 120 calories, 0g protein, 14g fat, 0g carbs
- Lemon Juice (1 tablespoon for dressing): 4 calories, 0g protein, 0g fat, 1g carbs

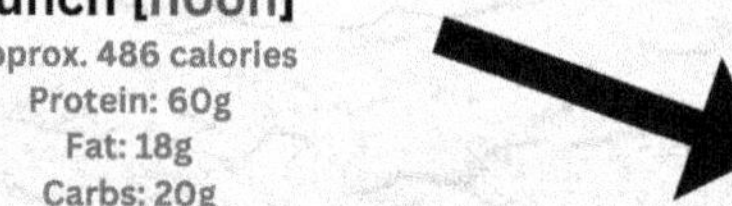

Afternoon Snack [3pm]

Approx. 200 calories
Protein: 9g
Fat: 9g
Carbs: 19g

- Hummus (2 tablespoons): 50 calories, 2g protein, 4g fat, 3g carbs
- Hard-Boiled Egg (1 large egg): 70 calories, 6g protein, 5g fat
- Mixed Berries (1/2 cup): 64 calories, 1g protein, 0g fat, 16g carbs

Dinner [6pm]

Approx. 567 calories
Protein: 45g
Fat: 34g
Carbs: 17g

- Baked Salmon (6 oz): 367 calories, 42g protein, 20g fat, 0g carbs
- Cauliflower Rice (1 cup): 25 calories, 1g protein, 0g fat, 5g carbs
- Steamed Broccoli (1 cup): 55 calories, 2g protein, 0g fat, 12g carbs
- Extra Virgin Olive Oil (1 tablespoon for cooking): 120 calories, 0g protein, 14g fat, 0g carbs

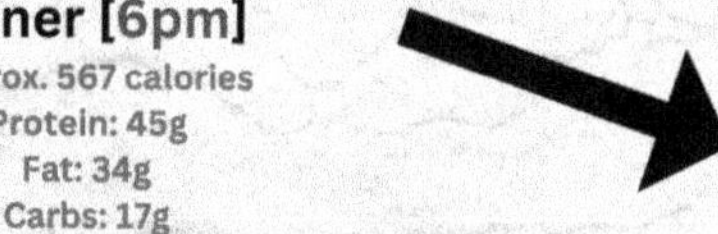

Evening Snack [8pm]

Approx. 150 calories
Protein: 14g
Fat: 2g
Carbs: 16g

- Cottage cheese (1/2 cup): 110 calories, 14g protein, 2g fat, 6g carbs
- Fresh pineapple chunks (1/2 cup): 40 calories, 0g protein, 0g fat, 10g carbs

TOTAL: 1,953 calories, 164g protein, 91g carbs, 93g fat

You would measure your food pre-cooked, input your measurements into the app, and do so with everything you eat. Don't worry about seasonings or sauces for now.

Breakfast [8am]
Approx. 350 calories
Protein: 17g
Fat: 41g
Carbs: 11g

- ***Scrambled Eggs (3 large eggs): 210 calories, 18g protein, 15g fat, 0g carbs***

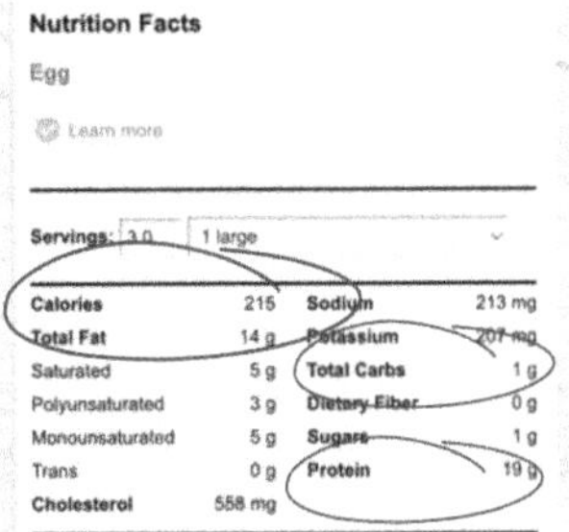

Nutrition Facts

Egg

Learn more

Servings: 3.0 | 1 large

Calories	215	Sodium	213 mg
Total Fat	14 g	Potassium	207 mg
Saturated	5 g	Total Carbs	1 g
Polyunsaturated	3 g	Dietary Fiber	0 g
Monounsaturated	5 g	Sugars	1 g
Trans	0 g	Protein	19 g
Cholesterol	558 mg		

Notice that these measurements aren't perfect, as the eggs that I used were slightly off from the eggs in the app. Try to keep the in-app measured food as close as possible to the actual food that you purchase.

- ***Avocado (1/2 avocado): 120 calories, 2g protein, 11g fat, 6g carbs***

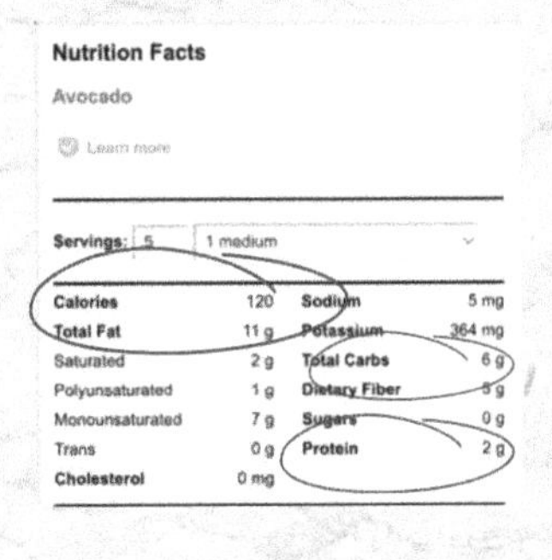

Nutrition Facts

Avocado

Learn more

Servings: .5 | 1 medium

Calories	120	Sodium	5 mg
Total Fat	11 g	Potassium	364 mg
Saturated	2 g	Total Carbs	6 g
Polyunsaturated	1 g	Dietary Fiber	5 g
Monounsaturated	7 g	Sugars	0 g
Trans	0 g	Protein	2 g
Cholesterol	0 mg		

Notice that these measurements are perfect, as the avocados I bought were the same ones in the app.

- ***Fresh Blueberries (1/2 cup): 20 calories, 0g protein, 0g fat, 5g carbs***

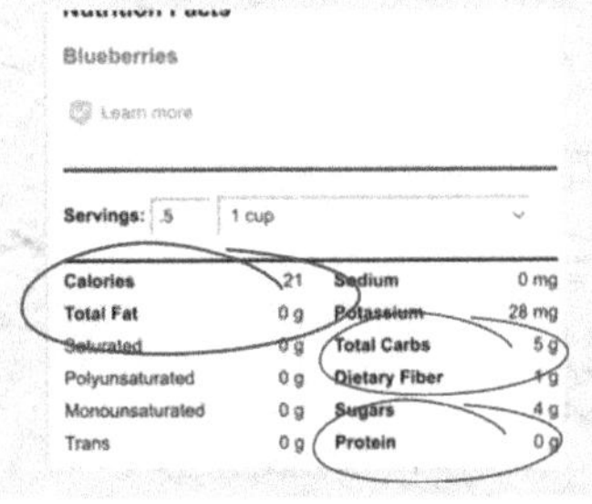

Blueberries

Learn more

Servings: .5 | 1 cup

Calories	21	Sodium	0 mg
Total Fat	0 g	Potassium	28 mg
Saturated	0 g	Total Carbs	5 g
Polyunsaturated	0 g	Dietary Fiber	1 g
Monounsaturated	0 g	Sugars	4 g
Trans	0 g	Protein	0 g

Notice that these measurements are near perfect, as the blueberries I bought weren't the exact same ones in the app.

EXAMPLE SCHEDULE

	Monday	Tuesday	Wednesday	Thursday	Friday	Saturday	Sunday
Breakfast	***Scrambled Eggs w/ Avocado and Blueberries:*** Approx. **300 calories** **Protein 18g** **Fat 20g** **Carbs 11g** • Scrambled Eggs (3 large eggs) • Avocado (1/2 avocado) • Fresh Blueberries (1/2 cup)	***Greek Yogurt Parfait:*** Approx. **350 calories** **Protein: 25g** **Fat: 10g** **Carbs: 45g** • 6 oz Greek yogurt • 1/2 cup fresh berries • 1/4 cup granola	***Peanut Butter Banana Smoothie:*** Approx. **370 calories** **Protein: 9g** **Fat: 18g** **Carbs: 39g** • 2 tbsp peanut butter • 1 banana • 1 cup almond milk	***Scrambled Eggs w/ Avocado and Blueberries:*** Approx. **350 calories** **Protein: 20g** **Fat: 41g** **Carbs: 11g** • Scrambled Eggs (3 large eggs) • Avocado (1/2 avocado) • Fresh Blueberries (1/2 cup)	***Cottage Cheese with Fruit:*** Approx. **310 calories** **Protein: 20g** **Fat: 5g** **Carbs: 45g** • 1 cup cottage cheese • Fresh mixed fruit (berries, melon)	***Breakfast Fruit Smoothie:*** Approx. **350 calories** **Protein: 15g** **Fat: 5g** **Carbs: 60g** • 1 ripe banana • 1 cup mixed berries (e.g., strawberries, blueberries, raspberries) • 6 oz Greek yogurt • 1 cup almond milk • 1 tablespoon honey	***Breakfast Burrito:*** Approx. **400 calories** **Protein: 20g** **Fat: 15g** **Carbs: 45g** • Scrambled Eggs (3 large eggs) • Black beans • salsa • gluten free tortilla
Snack	***Greek Yogurt w/ Almonds*** Approx. **180 calories** **Protein: 17g** **Fat: 4g** **Carbs: 8g** • Greek Yogurt (6 oz) • Almonds (1 oz, about 23 almonds)	***Pineapple Cottage Cheese*** Approx. **110 Calories** **Protein: 12g** **Fat: 1g** **Carbs: 14g** • 1/2 cup of cottage cheese • 1/2 cup of fresh pineapple chunks	***Apple with Peanut Butter*** Approx. **280 Calories** **Protein: 6g** **Fat: 18g** **Carbs: 24g** • 1 medium apple • 2 tablespoons of natural peanut butter	***Egg and Avocado*** Approx. **190 Calories** **Protein: 7g** **Fat: 15g** **Carbs: 6g** • 1 hard-boiled egg • 1/2 avocado	***Strawberry Greek Yogurt*** Approx. **220 Calories** **Protein: 15g** **Fat: 0g** **Carbs: 40g** • 6 ounces of Greek yogurt • 1/2 cup of fresh strawberries	***Almonds and Grapes*** Approx. **230 Calories** **Protein: 6g** **Fat: 14g** **Carbs: 20g** • 1 ounce (about 23) almonds • 1 cup of grapes	***Pear and Almond Butter*** Approx. **270 Calories** **Protein: 3g** **Fat: 21g** **Carbs: 17g** • 1 medium pear • 2 tablespoons of almond butter
Lunch	***Grilled Chicken w/ Brussel Sprouts and Sautéed Zucchini:*** Approx. **490 calories** **Protein: 63g** **Fat: 18g** **Carbs: 20g** • Grilled Chicken Breast (6 oz) • Roasted Brussels Sprouts (1 cup) • Sautéed Zucchini (1 cup) • Avocado Oil (1 tablespoon for cooking) • Lemon Juice (1 tablespoon for dressing)	***Taco bowl:*** Approx. **360 calories** **Protein: 54g** **Fat: 12g** **Carbs: 10g** 1 serving (bag) of Quest lime protein chips 3 oz of cooked 96%-4% lean ground beef 1 serving (28g) of fat free cheddar: 1 serving (2tbsp) salsa 1 serving (2tbsp) of light sour cream	***Salmon Salad:*** Approx. **340 calories** **Protein: 38g** **Fat: 16g** **Carbs: 10g** • 2 cups of mixed greens • 4oz baked salmon fillet • 1 serving (2 tbsp) of balsamic vinaigrette dressing • 1/4 cup cherry tomatoes • 1/4 cucumber, sliced	***Chicken Salad:*** Approx. **380 calories** **Protein: 47g** **Fat: 18g** **Carbs: 7g** • 2 cups of any lettuce/greens • 3oz grilled chicken breast: • 1 serving (2 tbsp) of light hidden valley ranch • 1 serving (28g) of fat free cheddar • 2 hard boiled eggs	***Mediterranean Quinoa Bowl:*** Approx. **430 calories** **Protein: 14g** **Fat: 22g** **Carbs: 44g** • 1 cup cooked quinoa • 3 oz grilled shrimp • 1/4 cup hummus • 1/4 cup diced cucumbers • 1/4 cup diced tomatoes • 1/4 cup diced red onions • 1 tablespoon olive oil and lemon juice dressing	***Chick-fil-a @ home:*** Approx. **500 calories** **Protein: 23g** **Fat: 25g** **Carbs: 46g** • Udis gluten free bun • Frozen fully cooked grilled chicken patty • 1 serving (85g) of Great Value Thin Cut French Fried Potatoes, 26 oz Bag (Frozen) • 1 serving/1 packet of chick-fil-a sauce	***Turkey and Avocado Wrap:*** Approx. **460 calories** **Protein: 30g** **Fat: 22g** **Carbs: 35g** • 4 oz turkey breast slices • 1 small gluten free tortilla or lettuce wrap • 1/2 avocado, sliced • 1/4 cup shredded carrots • 1/4 cup baby spinach leaves • 1 tablespoon Greek yogurt and Dijon mustard dressing

EXAMPLE SCHEDULE

	Monday	Tuesday	Wednesday	Thursday	Friday	Saturday	Sunday
Snack	**Rice Cakes with Almond Butter** **Calories: 180** **Protein: 4g** **Fat: 10g** **Carbs: 20g** • 2 rice cakes • 2 tablespoons of almond butter	**Turkey and Cheese** **Calories: 220** **Protein: 22g** **Fat: 13g** **Carbs: 3g** • 3 slices of turkey • 1 slice of cheese	**Chocolate Protein Shake** **Calories: 250** **Protein: 25g** **Fat: 6g** **Carbs: 25g** • 1 scoop of chocolate protein powder • 8 ounces of almond milk • 1 tablespoon of natural peanut butter	**Mixed Nuts** **Calories: 200** **Protein: 5g** **Fat: 17g** **Carbs: 8g** • 1 ounce of mixed nuts (walnuts, pecans, pine nuts, macadamia nuts, baruka, hazelnuts) • *AVOID using cashews, sunflower seeds, pumpkin seeds or peanuts	**Guacamole with Veggie Sticks** **Calories: 170** **Protein: 2g** **Fat: 14g** **Carbs: 8g** • 1/2 cup of guacamole • 1 cup of assorted veggie sticks (carrots, cucumber)	**Baby Carrots with Ranch** **Calories: 100** **Protein: 2g Fat: 7g** **Carbs: 6g** • 1 cup of baby carrots • 2 tablespoons of ranch dressing	**Chocolate Protein Shake** **Calories: 250** **Protein: 25g** **Fat: 6g** **Carbs: 25g** • 1 scoop of chocolate protein powder • 8 ounces of almond milk • 1 tablespoon of natural peanut butter
Dinner	**Salmon w/ Rice and Broccoli:** Approx. **550 calories** **Protein: 44g** **Fat: 34g** **Carbs: 17g** • Baked Salmon (6 oz) • Cauliflower Rice (1 cup) • Steamed Broccoli (1 cup) • Extra Virgin Olive Oil (1 tablespoon for cooking)	**Grilled Chicken with Sweet Potato and Steamed Asparagus:** Approx. **400 calories** **Protein: 40g** **Fat: 11g** **Carbs: 35g** • 6 oz grilled chicken breast • 1 medium baked sweet potato • 1 cup steamed asparagus • A sprinkle of black pepper	**Beef and Broccoli Stir-Fry:** Approx. **450 calories** **Protein: 38g** **Fat: 17g** **Carbs: 38g** • 5 oz lean beef strips • 1 cup broccoli florets • 1/2 cup cooked brown rice • 2 tablespoons low-sodium soy sauce	**Grilled Shrimp and Vegetable Skewers:** Approx. **320 calories** **Protein: 36g** **Fat: 15g** **Carbs: 14g** • 6 oz large shrimp • Assorted bell peppers, onions, and zucchini, skewered • 1 tablespoon olive oil and lemon juice marinade	**Beef and Black Bean Tacos:** Approx. **450 calories** **Protein: 30g** **Fat: 18g** **Carbs: 40g** • 4 oz ground beef • 1/2 cup black beans • Whole wheat or corn tortillas • Sliced lettuce, tomatoes, and a dollop of Greek yogurt	**Lemon Herb Grilled Chicken Thighs with Sweet Potatoes:** Approx. **380 calories** **Protein: 30g** **Fat: 15g** **Carbs: 30g** • 2 grilled chicken thighs • 1 baked sweet potato • A sprinkle of fresh herbs and a drizzle of lemon juice	**Baked Cod with Roasted Vegetables:** Approx. **380 calories** **Protein: 34g** **Fat: 16g** **Carbs: 28g** • 6 oz cod fillet • Assorted roasted vegetables (e.g., carrots, bell peppers, broccoli) • 1 tablespoon olive oil and lemon juice drizzle
Snack	**Dark Chocolate and Strawberries** **Calories: 120** **Protein: 2g** **Fat: 5g** **Carbs: 18g** • 1 ounce of dark chocolate • 1 cup of fresh strawberries	**Rice Cakes with Nutella** **Calories: 180** **Protein: 2g** **Fat: 8g** **Carbs: 25g** • 2 rice cakes • 2 tablespoons of Nutella	**Frozen Yogurt with Berries** **Calories: 150** **Protein: 5g** **Fat: 2g** **Carbs: 30g** • 1/2 cup of low-fat frozen yogurt • 1/2 cup of mixed berries	**Peanut Butter on Apple Slices** **Calories: 220** **Protein: 6g** **Fat: 16g** **Carbs: 12g** • 1 tablespoon of peanut butter • 1 medium apple, sliced	**Chocolate Protein Shake** **Calories: 250** **Protein: 25g** **Fat: 6g** **Carbs: 25g** • 1 scoop of chocolate protein powder • 8 ounces of almond milk • 1 tablespoon of natural peanut butter	**Fresh Fruit Salad** **Calories: 140** **Protein: 2g** **Fat: 1g** **Carbs: 30g** • A mixture of fresh fruit, such as berries, watermelon, cantaloupe, and pineapple.	**Frozen Banana Bites** **Calories: 130** **Protein: 1g** **Fat: 2g** **Carbs: 27g** • Sliced bananas dipped in chocolate and frozen

Balanced Dietary Principles:

A balanced diet is key to meeting your nutritional needs. It involves incorporating a variety of foods from different food groups in appropriate proportions. Aim to include more fruits, vegetables, lean proteins, and healthy fats in your meals. This variety ensures a diverse range of nutrients. It's also important to moderate your intake of certain carbohydrate types (really, carbs in general), added sugars, and unhealthy fats. As Americans, we should all immediately prioritize these *6 principles in order to balance our diet*:

1. **Eat less sugar (limit to 40g per day):**
    - We will go more in depth on sugar in Chapter 4, however it's of the utmost importance that you become aware of how much sugar you are consuming. Reduce the consumption of processed foods, sugary drinks, and desserts that contain high amounts of added sugars, which contributes to weight gain, chronic inflammation, and various health issues.

2. **Eat more vegetables (at least 2-3 cups per day):**
    - Vegetables are packed with essential vitamins, minerals, and fiber, supporting overall health, digestion, and immune function. Sadly, a staggering 90% of Americans fall short of consuming the daily recommended amount of vegetables.[4] Instead, this deficiency is compensated with an over-reliance on convenient highly-palatable carbohydrates and sugars in their diets. Many vegetables contain antioxidants that help combat oxidative stress, reduce inflammation, and protect against chronic diseases, including heart disease and certain cancers. Start replacing convenient carbs with equally convenient fruits and vegetables.

3. **Drink more water (at least 80-125 fluid ounces per day):**
    - Being hydrated is vital for maintaining proper bodily functions, including digestion, nutrient absorption, circulation, temperature regulation, and joint lubrication. Drinking water can help suppress appetite, enhance metabolism, and support healthy weight management by replacing sugary beverages. Sadly, the average American only drinks about 44 fluid ounces of water per day - far below the recommended 101 fluid ounces (about 13 cups) per day for men and 74 fluid ounces (about 9 cups) per day for women.[5]

4. **Eat more protein (at least 80-120 grams per day):**
    - Protein is crucial for tissue development and repair, playing an essential role in supporting muscle growth and recovery. Maintaining an adequate protein intake is vital to ensure these processes function optimally. Additionally, protein-rich foods contribute to satiety, reducing cravings and assisting in appetite regulation. This can facilitate weight management and reduce the likelihood of overeating. Proteins consist of various amino acids, including essential amino acids that the human body cannot create independently. Hence, a sufficient intake of dietary protein, encompassing a variety of protein sources, is necessary to obtain an adequate supply of essential amino acids.
    - *Note that essential amino acids can easily be supplemented with supplements like protein powders, however there is still the necessity for a "whole-foods" priority for our sources of protein.

5. **Prioritize cooking at home over dining out:**
    - Preparing meals at home offers several advantages for your health and well-being. It also saves you a ton of money in the end. Whoever told you that eating healthy is more expensive is half correct: it's more expensive to buy healthier ingredients than cheaper processed ingredients, true. However, it is far more expensive to buy convenient unhealthy fast food than it is to buy healthier ingredients and prepare the food yourself. Ultimately, when you take control of your food preparation, you have the power to choose wholesome ingredients and control portion sizes. Cooking at home allows you to prioritize nutrition by incorporating a variety of nutrient-dense foods into your meals. Additionally, it gives you the opportunity to experiment with different flavors and cooking techniques, making your dining experience more enjoyable and fulfilling. Cooking at home more frequently fosters a healthier relationship with food, improves your culinary skills, and more importantly saves money that you can then reinvest back into your healthy lifestyle.

6. **Avoid Excess Anti-Nutrients and Seed Oils**
    - We'll delve into this topic further in Chapter 6, but it's essential to emphasize the importance of avoiding certain anti-nutrients - like lectins, oxalates, and phytates, along with steering clear of harmful seed oils. These compounds, found in various foods, have the potential to disrupt nutrient absorption and digestion. Many of the anti-nutrients we'll discuss in Chapter 6 are naturally occurring defensive chemicals in certain foods, primarily specific plants. Being mindful of your consumption of foods rich in these anti-nutrients and avoiding detrimental seed oils can significantly enhance your nutrient absorption and promote a healthier gut.

Portion Control

Discovering the delicate art of portion control and embracing the concept of satiety (feeling full) is pivotal in cultivating a positive relationship with food. It extends beyond mere measurements, and encompasses our satisfaction and hunger levels. When we understand the significance of portion control and making mindful choices about the foods we consume, we can achieve a greater sense of satiety, reduce cravings for unhealthy options, and enhance our dietary discipline.

It's important to note that when your stomach rumbles, it doesn't mean that you're starving or even necessarily hungry; in fact, it's more than likely just your stomach begging for sugar. Without delving into it too deeply, try to understand that the feelings of being hungry and starving are very, very different, and you will survive that ultimate feeling of "hunger" when you start shifting your dietary choices.

Developing a conscious awareness of what and how much we eat is fundamental to practicing portion control effectively. By paying attention to our hunger cues and adopting mindful eating habits, we can make informed decisions about what we eat. The biggest decision that we should make as Americans is choosing *how much to eat.* Start eating more slowly, savoring each bite, and allow your body time to register fullness and satisfaction.

Portion control is instrumental in maintaining a healthy weight and supporting sustainable healthy habits. It is crucial to manage your portion sizes so that you can achieve a balance between energy intake and energy expenditure. This helps prevent the overconsumption of calories, which is why we get overweight.

At first, you will feel less full from diminishing your portions, but as you continue to eat in smaller portions, your stomach will literally shrink and you will not expect/seem to need the big portions you once expected/thought you needed.

A well-balanced diet is the cornerstone of clean eating and sustaining healthy eating habits. It entails incorporating a diverse array of clean-sourced and natural nutrients into our meals. Based on our anatomy, human beings are biologically hardwired as "opportunistic omnivores" meaning our bodies are really good at utilizing anything and everything for fuel. Though this is true, it is important to note that our bodies do prefer and prioritize certain nutrients over others. It is also important to note that we all have different body types, and no one human responds the same to all food groups. We all have our own unique tolerances and degrees of tolerances to different food types and different food quantities. As a result, *there is no "one perfect formula" when it comes to constructing a universal diet for anyone and everyone to follow.* However, there are universal truths when it comes to nutrition, and by realizing these universal truths it allows the individual to subjectively calibrate their unique dietary needs in accordance to base laws of nutrition.

Understanding the basic laws of nutrition empowers you with the knowledge to make informed choices about the foods you eat. In simply knowing about the importance of macronutrients, the principles of a balanced diet, and the importance of portion control, you can begin to take control of your health and well-being. When we implement these strategies, we can develop a healthier relationship with food, reduce cravings for sugary and unhealthy options, and achieve an 80/20 balanced diet. In Chapter 3, we will breakdown how digestion works so we can become aware of what exactly is happening in our bodies when we fuel it.

Chapter 3

How Digestion Works In Laymen's Terms

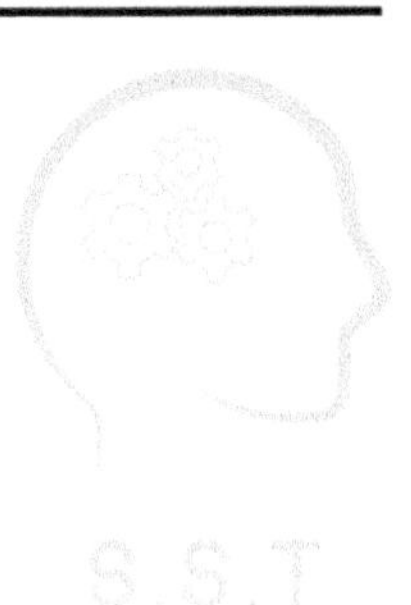

Digestion is a complex process that allows our bodies to break down food into smaller molecules that can then be absorbed and used for energy. Having worked with countless clients, I've come to understand the importance of them having a solid grasp on how digestion works in order for them to become self sustained in making healthy dietary decisions.

Without going too in depth on the complex relationship between the circulatory system and the digestive system, just know that the heart is crucial for pumping blood and blood is the transporter of all of our biochemicals and nutrients. And when we are chronically inflamed, it constricts the circulation of our blood flow, causes our hearts to pump harder (hence high blood pressure), and thus diminishes the overall effectiveness of our body's circulation.

The heart serves as the central pump, constantly contracting and relaxing to propel blood throughout the body. Arteries, veins, and capillaries form a network of blood vessels that transport oxygen, nutrients, hormones, and immune cells to different tissues and organs. When our body is chronically inflamed and lacks proper circulation, it cannot transport our necessary biochemicals as thoroughly, subsequently degrading our health. Plus, when we're overweight, our heart has to work that much harder in order to combat against how heavy we are in tandem with chronic inflammation and poor circulation. The heavier we are, the harder the heart has to work.

In this chapter, we will focus on digestion, but it is important to preface the importance of digestion with regards to the decreasing of inflammation that ultimately leads to better circulation - which is the key to longevity and being healthy.

Let's think of digestion using a basic analogy. Though our digestive system is more like a plumbing system, we will compare our digestive system to a well-coordinated team of workers in a factory. Just as each worker in the factory has a specific role in the production line, our digestive organs have distinct functions in breaking down food and extracting nutrients.

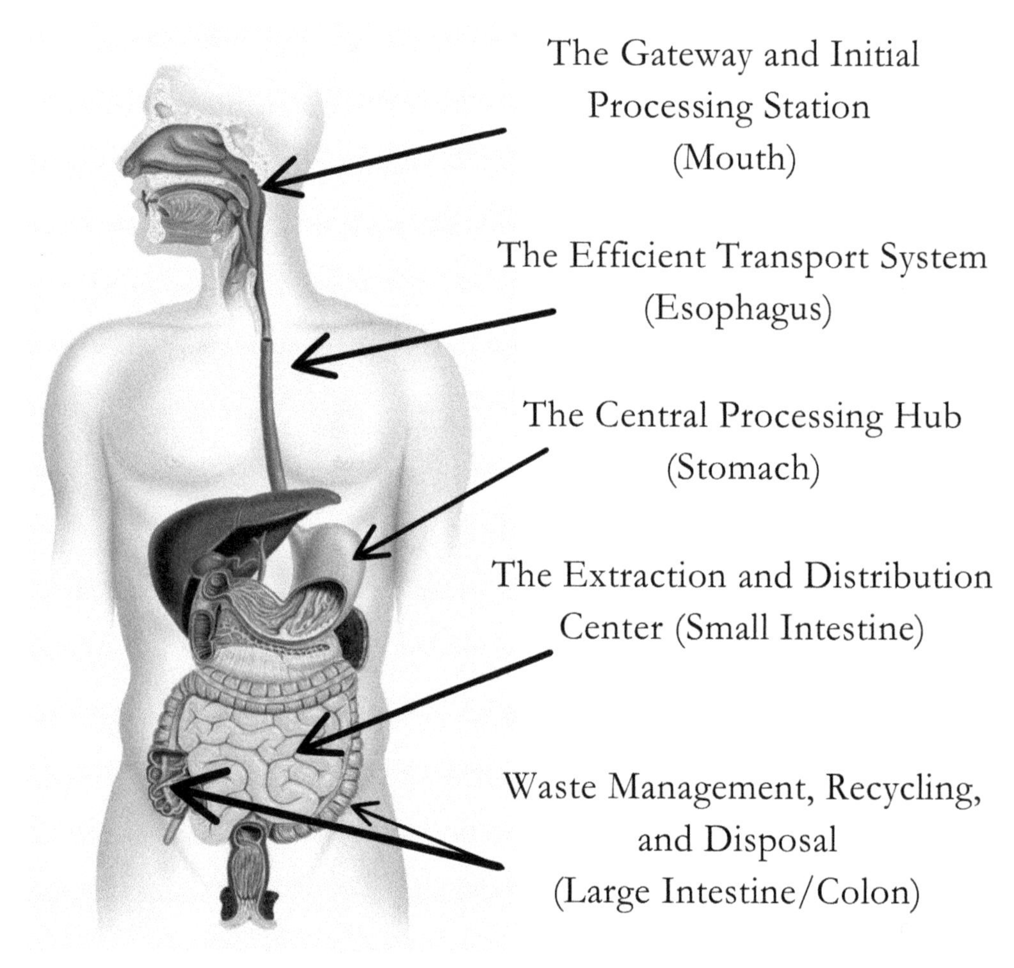

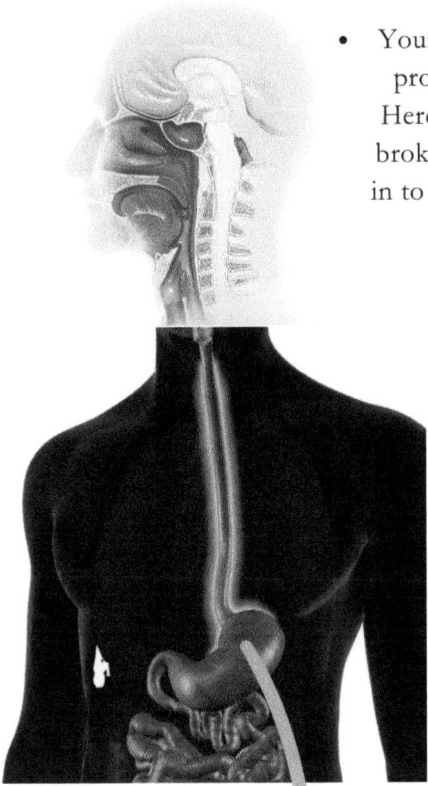

The Gateway and Initial Processing Station (Mouth):

- Your mouth serves as the gateway and initial processing station of the digestive system. Here, the food you consume is mechanically broken down by chewing, and saliva is mixed in to begin the process of chemical digestion.

The Efficient Transport System (Esophagus):

- The esophagus acts as an efficient transport system, carrying the chewed food from your mouth to your stomach. It accomplishes this by rhythmic muscle contractions, known as peristalsis, which propel the food downward in a coordinated manner.

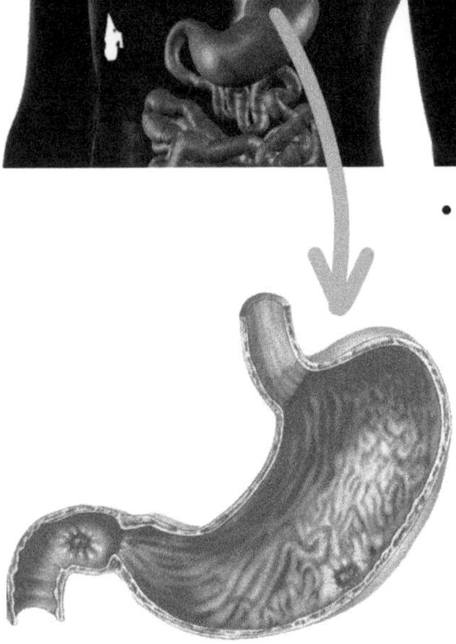

The Central Processing Hub (Stomach):

- When the food reaches the stomach, it has reached the central processing hub. Here, the stomach muscles contract and mix the food with digestive juices, including hydrochloric acid and certain enzymes. The acid helps break down any bacteria, while specific enzymes start breaking down carbs, proteins, and fats into their smaller forms (carbs broken down into glucose, proteins into amino acids, and fats into fatty acids), though they are fully broken down and absorbed in the small intestine.

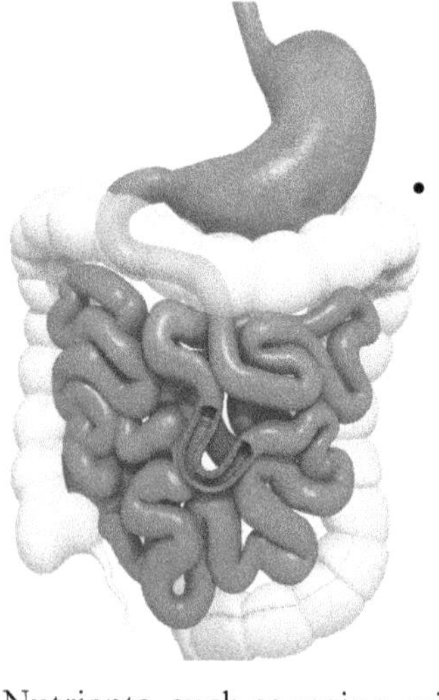

The Extraction and Distribution Center
(Small Intestine):

- The partially digested food then enters the small intestine, which acts as an extraction and distribution center. It receives additional digestive enzymes from the pancreas and bile from the liver and gallbladder. These substances further break down carbs, proteins, and fats into their smaller building blocks, which can then be absorbed by the body. It is in the small intestine where carbs, protein, and fats are fully broken down and is where 95% of nutrient absorption should occur.[1] Nutrients, such as amino acids from protein, glucose from carbs, fatty acids from fats, vitamins, and minerals, are absorbed into the bloodstream through the small intestine's specialized lining (hence the important of our gut lining). The small intestine is responsible for the majority of nutrient absorption, and once the nutrients are absorbed into the bloodstream, they are transported throughout the body and to the cells where cellular respiration takes place. Cellular respiration is how cells convert the food we eat into energy.

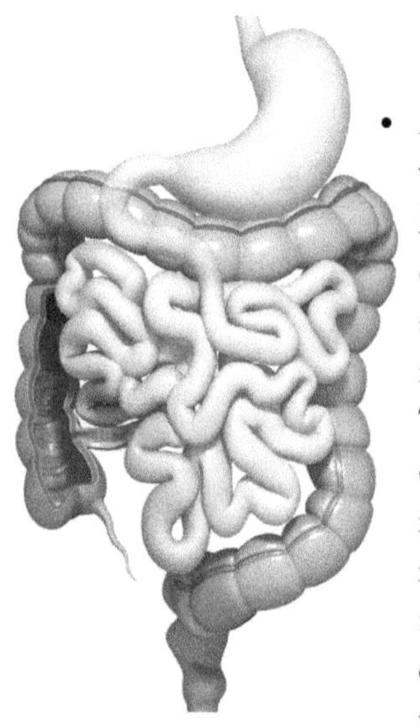

Waste Management, Recycling, and Disposal
(Large Intestine/Colon):

- After the nutrients have been extracted, the remaining waste material, along with undigested fibers and other indigestible components, enters the large intestine or colon. The colon's main role is to digest fiber and absorb water and electrolytes from the waste material, making it more solid and preparing it for elimination. The colon (large intestine) is also home to a diverse community of microorganisms, known as gut microbiota (also known as a communal gut microbiome), which aids in the fermentation and further breakdown of undigested fibers and other compounds in the final production of waste. Once these residual components are made into waste, they are then disposed of out the anus as poop.

In the intricate dance of energy production within our cells, several key players come together to ensure the smooth flow of healthy metabolism. There are two primary players, however, which are *insulin* and *glucose.*

As described, cellular respiration is how cells convert the food that we eat into energy for the body. Without explaining the full bioenergetic reality of what occurs during cellular respiration, simply think about it like this: when food reaches our small intestine, it is broken down into its smallest components; proteins into amino acids, fats into fatty acids, and carbs into a particular sugar known as glucose. When these smaller compounds leave the small intestine and enter the bloodstream, the blood begins transporting these essential nutrients throughout the body in order to be absorbed and used for various uses.

Unlike amino acids and fatty acids (which are easily absorbed by our cells), glucose cannot be absorbed by our cells without having some form of assistance. This is literally what insulin is for: to help glucose get into the cell membrane so that it can be used as energy. Think of insulin as the key that unlocks the cell to allow glucose to enter. Once glucose enters the cell, it is then broken down and converted into energy. Remember, glucose is simply the most broken down form of a carbohydrate known as a sugar, so blood sugar levels only spike when we consume carbs. Otherwise, when we only consume amino acids via proteins and fatty acids via fats, our blood sugar levels remain relatively low. This is why it is so important to start your day with high protein foods and healthy-fat foods rather than high carbohydrate foods; to minimize blood sugar spikes and sustain energy levels throughout the day. Though our cells prefer to utilize glucose (carbs) for energy production, our bodies are able to utilize protein and fats as well - namely fats, as mentioned before, during prolonged periods of absent glucose.

Insulin is a hormone produced by the pancreas. Insulin acts as a master regulator, orchestrating the uptake, use, and storage of glucose from the bloodstream and into our cells. This means that anytime we consume carbohydrates, insulin is released, signaling cells to open their doors and allow glucose to enter. Without insulin, we could not use glucose. Without insulin, we would not be able to utilize carbs as energy.

This glucose is then utilized as a primary source of energy or stored for later use. If we consume too much glucose (which 90%+ of Americans seem to do) then we excessively raise our insulin levels which, without going too deep into it, causes metabolic dysfunction - which simply means the disregulation of how we digest and process food (namely carbs). Too much insulin is bad for the body, and it in combination with too much glucose ultimately leads to *metabolic dysfunction* - specifically insulin resistance and eventually type 2 diabetes.

Insulin resistance is a condition in which the body's cells become less responsive to the effects of insulin on glucose to where "the key doesn't fit" the cell anymore. It is essentially the body building a tolerance to higher and higher blood sugar levels, meaning it requires more and more insulin to push glucose into the cell. In the context of cellular respiration, insulin resistance disrupts the normal flow of glucose into the cells, leading to less uptake/usage of glucose in the blood and a decrease in energy metabolism. This simply means that glucose cannot efficiently enter the cells, resulting in reduced energy production. Due to this, the cells are unable to take in the glucose from the blood, leaving them there and leading to *elevated blood sugar levels.*

Moreover, insulin resistance initiates a cascade of metabolic disturbances that go beyond its immediate impact on glucose regulation and the cell's responsiveness to insulin's signals. When the pancreas responds to produce higher levels of insulin in an attempt to overcome such resistance, this heightened insulin presence in the bloodstream can instigate a pro-inflammatory state, fostering chronic inflammation.

Another key component to our metabolic health is our gut microbiome, which is primarily located in the large intestine (colon). The gut microbiome is a community of microorganisms ("bacteria") that is often referred to as the "brain of your stomach" and dignifies the idea of 'you are what you eat'. The gut microbiome is super significant for your digestive and general health. These bacteria assist in a process called fermentation that affects undigested carbohydrates, fiber, and other compounds that reach the large intestine due to not being fully processed in the small intestine. This is primarily due to anti-nutrients, high-processed foods, and excess food being digested (we will discuss fermentation more in depth later). Essentially, when compounds like yeast are not enzymatically broken down in the small intestine to then undergo cellular respiration, they are instead passed onto the large intestine to undergo digestion via fermentation. While fermentation is a natural and beneficial process, it can lead to complications when the body is chronically fermenting inflammatory foods.

In addition to their role in fermentation, certain bacteria and cells in the intestines contribute to the production of serotonin, a neurotransmitter known for its role in mood regulation, appetite, sleep, and other important functions. Remarkably, 90-95% of serotonin is created in the cells of the intestinal wall, meaning nearly all of our brain and body's serotonin is made in our gut.[2] This serotonin is subsequently released into the bloodstream and travels to the brain, playing a vital role in regulating mood, appetite, and sleep. However, when the body is in a state of chronic inflammation or malnourishment, the production of serotonin becomes compromised, leading to an inadequate supply for maintaining optimal health functions like a healthy mood, an appropriate appetite, and quality sleep. The intricate connection between the gut microbiota and serotonin production highlights the intimate influence of dietary choices on mental and emotional well-being.

The modern American diet, often laden with excessive amounts of processed foods, added sugars, and unhealthy fats, triggers inflammation within the gut. This inflammation disrupts the delicate balance in both the small and large intestines. In the small intestine, it disrupts the production of serotonin and nutrient absorption. In the large intestine, it disturbs the gut microbiome, leading to an overabundance of fermentation. Excessive fermentation in the large intestine results in discomforting symptoms such as gas, bloating, and even contributes to conditions like leaky gut syndrome.

It is important to note that the impact of excessive consumption of inflammatory foods, the subsequent disruption of serotonin production, and over-fermentation in the intestines can vary from person to person. While some individuals may possess a higher tolerance for these foods, others may experience more pronounced discomfort and disturbances within their digestive system. Either way, we should all be more mindful of how inflammatory our diets can become.

A concept worth noting that deserves its own entire book is a concept known as intermittent fasting. Intermittent fasting is a practical way to give your digestive tract a break, regulate your food intake, and minimize unnecessary snacking. This approach involves cycling between eating and fasting periods, with fasting windows typically lasting from 14 to 18 hours. During the fasting phase, you abstain from food and only consume your daily meals within a condensed time frame of 6 to 10 hours.

Intermittent fasting provides a practical means for individuals to cultivate mindfulness about their dietary choices. By limiting the eating window, intermittent fasting reduces the likelihood of impulsive snacking and encourages a more conscious approach to meal planning. Not only this, but the advantages of intermittent fasting go beyond just curbing your eating habits; it has a positive impact on your digestive and metabolic health. The benefits of intermittent fasting can help with metabolic adaptations, such as re-sensitizing our insulin sensitivity and improving our blood sugar regulation.

It should be noted that intermittent fasting affects men and women differently, so ladies should be more cautious when implementing fasting into their weekly routine. Without diving too deep into it, I advise my female clients who want to intermittent fast to limit their intermittent fasting to 3x per week, but before you embark on it you should do some due diligence in researching or consulting with a professional first. Again, fasting deserves its own book and there is plenty of material out there for you to educate yourself on fasting if that's an avenue you're interested in exploring.

As discussed, frequent or excessive carbohydrate consumption can lead to insulin resistance, disrupting the balance of blood sugar and impairing metabolic health. Intermittent fasting provides a break from continuous carbohydrate intake, allowing the body to reset its insulin sensitivity. During fasting periods, the body shifts to utilizing stored energy, primarily from fats. Think of all the fat on your body - that fat is energy waiting to be used. Now this is oversimplifying it, but if you can sensitize your body to using the fat stores you have stored, then you can use that energy instead of having to eat carbs. This process helps lower overall insulin levels and improve the body's responsiveness to insulin whenever we do eat. As a result, blood sugar remains stable, and the risk of insulin resistance, pre-diabetes, and type 2 diabetes effectively decreases.

Moreover, fasting can have a positive impact on the gut microbiome. While fermentation is a natural process (as we will discuss in chapter 4), excessive consumption of inflammatory foods can lead to over-fermentation and gastrointestinal discomfort. Intermittent fasting provides the gut with periods of rest, allowing it to recover from the constant influx of food.

Fasting not only gives your digestive system a much-needed break, but it can also be a game-changer in simplifying your eating habits. By adopting a shortened eating window, you'll naturally consume fewer snacks, and meal planning becomes more straightforward.

Through envisioning the intricate process of digestion via our simplified analogy, you attain a deeper comprehension of the intriguing journey that food undergoes to transform into the energy your body requires. Prioritizing a well-balanced diet, encompassing whole, minimally processed foods, and remaining mindful of the influence of inflammatory foods on gut health, becomes imperative. Collaborating with healthcare professionals can provide personalized guidance in making informed dietary decisions. However, you can remedy enough dietary changes to become healthier without needing to depend on any professional by becoming informed yourself about the very underlying variables said professionals are measuring.

Remember, tending to the needs of your digestive system serves as the cornerstone of optimal health and sustainable vitality. I always emphasize to my clients the importance of incorporating natural whole foods, particularly more fruits and veggies, into our diet and the invaluable benefits they offer - especially in regard to our gut health. This is particularly crucial considering that the majority of us fall short in consuming an adequate amount of either fruits or veggies. By prioritizing the substitution of sugary snacks with wholesome fruit or veggie options, we can begin replacing habitual behaviors with intentional actions. In Chapter 4, this will become even more prevalent as we begin to explore the unsweet truth about sugar.

Chapter 4

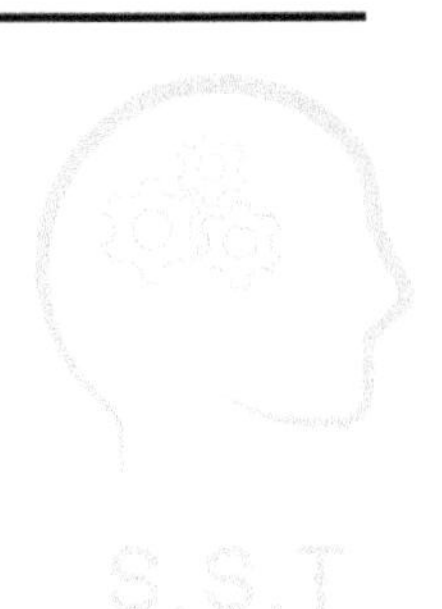

The Unsweet Truth About Sugar

In today's modern diet, sugar has become universally accepted as a necessary evil, slithering its way into a wide array of foods and beverages. While a moderate amount of sugar can be enjoyed as part of a balanced diet, excessive sugar consumption has been linked to numerous health concerns.

In this chapter, we will delve into the reasons why it is recommended that we all limit our sugar intake to less than 40 grams per day. When we understand the impact of sugar on our health and explore practical strategies to reduce its consumption, we can take control of our diets and promote the absolute best version of ourselves.

There are technically 3 types of sugars: glucose, fructose, and galactose. Glucose (as we've gone over a million times at this point) comes from carbs and is the body's preferred energy source. Fructose and galactose, however, are a little different. Fructose comes primarily from fruit, but is also found in some vegetables like bell peppers and squash, as well as natural sweeteners like honey or agave. Galactose is the simple sugar found in dairy like milk and cheese. Sugar, as you know it, is really just a combination of fructose + glucose, which is really known as *sucrose* or table sugar.

The bitter reality of excessive sugar intake has deep roots in human history. Throughout centuries, sugar consumption has progressively evolved, leading us down a path that includes the rise of processed sugars like *high fructose corn syrup*. For our ancestors, sugar in the form of fructose was a rare and treasured commodity, reserved for special occasions and indulgences. However, as technology advanced and food production became more efficient, sugar became more accessible and the main affordable commodity for the masses.

Unfortunately, the widespread availability of sugar also brought about a detrimental shift in our eating habits. The introduction of highly processed sugars into our food supply, such as high fructose corn syrup, has had a profound impact on our health. These sugars are anti-nutritious and are often added to foods and beverages to enhance flavor and prolong shelf life. This shift towards processed sugars has led to a dramatic increase in sugar consumption, contributing to the obesity epidemic and a host of modern diseases.

As mentioned before, when we consume high amounts of glucose it rapidly enters the bloodstream, causing blood sugar spikes and triggering the release of the hormone insulin. Fructose, however, does not signal for insulin release and instead signals for other hormones like leptin and ghrelin, which are responsible for appetite and hunger cues. A doctor would say something like "fructose attenuates postprandial suppression of ghrelin" which is a fancy way of saying fructose decreases the body's ability to suppress hunger after eating. And that's because ghrelin is the hormone that tells your body that you're hungry, where leptin tells your body that you're full. Without going too deep into it, fructose increases ghrelin and decreases leptin, and is like a drug that essentially tells your body to search for more fructose (hence a 'rumbling stomach' as alluded to earlier) and slows down your body's ability to "not be hungry" - causing you to still feel hungry after eating.

Not only this, but a big difference between glucose and fructose is how they are metabolized by the body. Where glucose is metabolized and sent into the bloodstream to be used as needed, fructose is metabolized and sent directly to the liver to either be turned into glucose or triglycerides. Some of the fructose is converted into glucose to be used as energy, stored as glucose in the form of glycogen, or converted into fat and stored as triglycerides (making you fat; this is how carbs/sugar make you fat and not dietary fats). This can contribute to an increase in fat accumulation in the liver. In fact, excessive sugar has been implicated in the rising prevalence of non-alcoholic fatty liver disease (NAFLD), with approximately 25% of American adults and 10% of American children being affected.[1]

This is a significant departure from the past, where the only sufferers of fatty liver disease less than 100 years ago were typically alcoholics - which is why the more recent condition is named non-alcoholic fatty liver disease to distinguish it from alcohol-related liver disease. Sadly, liver diseases related to excessive alcohol consumption and an overindulgence in sugar have become significant health concerns in the United States. Depending on the region and population, the prevalence of alcoholic liver disease can vary in relation to the prevalence of sugar in the regions' diet, compounding the effects of regular and chronic alcohol use that leads to alcoholic liver disease. We will discuss the toxic effects of alcohol more in depth in the next chapter.

NAFLD, on the other hand, has seen a rising prevalence in recent years and can affect individuals who do not consume alcohol - like children. It is primarily associated with factors such as obesity, insulin resistance, and metabolic dysfunction, which are all consequences of excessive sugar intake.

Understanding the detrimental effects of excess sugar in the body underscores the importance of reducing its consumption - the effects being fructose's implication on hunger cues and glucose's impact on insulin and insulin resistance. Just taking the first step of decreasing sugar intake helps mitigate its overall consequences. Sugar is also a vasoconstrictor, meaning it tightens our blood vessels, so decreasing its intake will help decrease constricting inflammation and promote improved circulation. To support this process, it is crucial to prioritize drinking water and consuming nutrient-dense foods that provide essential vitamins, minerals, fiber, and other nourishing elements. This approach supports an improved inflammatory and circulatory response.

I often remind my clients that an inflamed body coupled with poor posture is like a swollen hose with a kink in it - hindering the flow of water. From a biomechanical standpoint, we aim to train the body to become more resilient, like a kink-resistant hose, allowing essential nutrients, vitamins, and minerals to flow freely throughout the system. From a nutritional perspective, the focus is on learning to make better food choices to reduce the bloated and constricted nature of the system. When the body is less swollen and inflammation is minimized, the circulation of vital nutrients becomes more efficient. Sugar acts as a blood-constricting antagonist to this goal, perpetuating chronic inflammation and hindering the body's natural healing processes.

Reducing sugar intake can be a challenging task, primarily due to the prevalence of hidden sugars in processed foods and beverages. Many manufacturers use various names for added sugars, making it difficult for consumers to identify them on ingredient lists. When we become familiar with these aliases and develop the habit of carefully reading food labels, we can make more informed choices and opt for lower-sugar alternatives. Ideally, you won't have to even worry about this list because, in an ideal world, you would be getting all of your fructose-based sugar from fruits and fruits alone.

Common Hidden Sugars

Be aware of these hidden sugars and their alternative names. In doing so, you can become more adept at identifying them on food labels.

1. **High Fructose Corn Syrup:**
- This highly processed sweetener is derived from corn and is commonly found in many processed foods, including sodas, fruit drinks, baked goods, and condiments.
2. **Dextrose:**
- Dextrose is a form of glucose derived from cornstarch and is often used as a sweetener and a food additive in various processed foods, such as candies, desserts, and energy bars.
3. **Fructose:**
- Fructose is a natural sugar found in fruits, but it is also used as an added sweetener in various processed foods, such as sodas, fruit-flavored drinks, and sweetened snacks.
4. **Sucrose:**
- Sucrose is the scientific name for table sugar, which is a combination of glucose and fructose. It is widely used in baking, desserts, sweetened beverages, and processed foods.
5. **Maltose:**
- Maltose is a sugar composed of two glucose molecules and is often used as a sweetener in processed foods, such as cereals, malted beverages, and certain sauces.
6. **Syrups:**
- Different types of syrups, such as maple syrup, agave syrup, and rice syrup, are commonly used as sweeteners in processed foods, baked goods, and breakfast cereals.
7. **Molasses:**
- Molasses is a thick, dark syrup produced during the sugar refining process and is often used as a sweetener in baked goods, marinades, and condiments.

Reducing sugar intake doesn't mean depriving ourselves of all sweetness. It's about adopting healthier habits and finding alternatives that satisfy our taste buds while minimizing the inflammatory effects of excessive sugar consumption.

Here are some practical strategies I recommend to my clients to help them cut back on sugar:

1. **Opt for whole, unprocessed foods**: Fresh fruits should be the primary source of your fructose-based sugar intake. These natural foods provide essential nutrients without the added sugars found in many processed options.
2. **Be mindful of sugary beverages**: Sugary drinks like soda, fruit juices, and sweetened coffee or tea can contribute a significant amount of hidden sugar to your daily intake. Opt for water, black coffee, unsweetened tea, or infused water with fresh fruits for a refreshing and hydrating alternative.
3. **Read food labels**: Familiarize yourself with the sugar content listed on food labels and choose products with lower sugar amounts. Pay attention to serving sizes, as sometimes products may appear to have less sugar, but the portion size may be smaller.
4. **Prepare meals at home**: By cooking your meals from scratch, you have control over the ingredients and can limit the amount of added sugars. Experiment with herbs, spices, and natural sweeteners like cinnamon or vanilla extract to enhance flavors without relying on excessive sugar.
5. **Limit processed and packaged foods**: Processed snacks, desserts, and pre-packaged meals often contain hidden sugars. Opt for homemade alternatives or choose snacks that are low in added sugars, such as nuts, seeds, or, you guessed it, fresh fruit.
6. **Gradually reduce added sugars**: Start by gradually decreasing the amount of sugar you add to your beverages or recipes. The goal is to maintain less than 40g of sugar per day. Over time, your taste buds will adjust, and you'll find that you need less sugar to satisfy your cravings.

Remember, small changes can yield significant results, and over time, your taste buds will adapt to lower sugar levels.
Excessive sugar consumption poses risks to our health, including obesity, diabetes, and heart disease. Adhering to the scientific recommended limits of 38 grams of sugar per day for men and 25 grams per day for women[2] will significantly contribute to a healthier lifestyle, though I generally use the rule of thumb of consuming less than 40g for the average American adult.

Through awareness, mindful choices, and discipline, the strategies listed will help you in reducing your sugar intake and enjoy the natural sweetness of a balanced diet.

Chapter 5

Fermentability of Foods: The Effects of Alcohol and Fermentable Sugars

For the majority of modern Americans, there is a struggle with gut inflammation, and we are now starting to understand why. In the context of chronic gut inflammation, it's important to understand the "fermentability of foods" as some foods undergo a processed called *fermentation* in the large intestine (colon). Fermentable foods are those that are broken down by bacteria in your colon, leading to gas and digestive discomfort. Without scientifically explaining what exactly this means, just know that alcohol and excessive sugar (which we'll generalize as fermentable sugars) cause an over stimulation of the liver and colon, which exacerbates overall inflammation.

The modern American diet therefore causes the large intestine to do more work than it otherwise ever would. The colon's preferred source for fermentation is dietary fiber, particularly *soluble fiber.* Any other substances reaching the colon may disrupt the gut microbiota and cause digestive unrest.

Think of it like this: the small intestine is where 95% of digestion should occur,[1] and the other 5% should occur in the colon, and the primary food the colon prefers is fiber - particularly soluble fiber, which we will discuss. We will also discuss how excess fermentable sugars like fructose and alcohol cause an over-fermentation in the intestines while simultaneously destroying the intestinal lining.

With that said, neither of our intestines like alcohol or excessive sugar.

In this chapter, we will go over the differences between fermentable and non-fermentable foods and why these terms are important to know. Alcohol (also known as ethanol) is a specific fermented substance with a long history that causes unnecessary inflammation. While alcohol, or ethanol, doesn't ferment in our body (as it is already fermented), its effects disturb how fermentation occurs in our colon. The main negative impact that alcohol has on our body is how it destroys our liver and gut lining - subsequently toxifying our body in the process. Eliminating alcohol alone from your diet will lead to life-changing results - although this may be difficult considering over 60% of American adults admit to drinking regularly.[2] When we sip on alcohol, it swiftly enters our bloodstream and transforms into a toxic compound called acetaldehyde, which triggers the not-so-pleasant effects of intoxicative inflammation within the body.

Outside of alcohol, fermentable sugars (namely excessive fructose) play a primary role in exacerbating gut inflammation. These sugars, when fermented in the colon, stimulate the growth of bad gut bacteria, potentially leading to discomfort or digestive issues. Given how bad both alcohol and fermentable sugars are for the body (namely the liver and gut), it is easiest to classify the effects of both as being very similar. In that alcohol and excessive sugar both destroy our gut lining and build fat around our organs (namely the liver, hence the association between alcohol, and now fructose, with fatty liver disease). Being mindful of the effects of both alcohol and added sugars on gut inflammation allows us to make healthier nutritional choices that restore digestive health and rebuild the integrity of our body's digestive tract.

Fermentable Foods

Fruits and vegetables are the primary fermentable foods that you should be consuming - as they are dense in soluble fiber. Soluble fiber is what our body wants and is a vital component for gut health, as it aids in forming soft, well-formed stools, promoting healthy digestion. Insoluble fiber, on the other hand, cannot be processed by our body, which then contributes to loose stools and less beneficial digestive health.

This choice becomes especially important when dealing with gut inflammation. Certain fermentable foods like whole grains and corn are full of fiber - just not the right type of fiber. These highly fermentable foods can exacerbate inflammation in the gut. Hence the essential need to exercise caution when including them in your diet. Instead of avoiding all fermentable foods, prioritize soluble fiber over insoluble fiber, and incorporate more fruits and vegetables.

Though certain fermentable grains (wheat, corn, beans, oats, etc.) can bring some value as a part of a balanced diet, it's important to approach them with caution if you're already dealing with gut inflammation - which the majority of us are.

Fermentable foods like fruits and vegetables often have a lower energy density, providing fewer calories per gram compared to non-fermentable foods. This can be beneficial for weight management, as they can help create a feeling of fullness without contributing excessive calories. However, their fermentable nature may stimulate the growth of bacteria in the large intestine, potentially exacerbating gut inflammation and leading to poor digestion. Therefore avoiding certain highly fermentable foods (like whole grains, particularly wheat) is important for losing weight and decreasing overall inflammation. With that said, certain highly fermentable foods (like fruits and veggies) need to stay in your diet no matter what. So it becomes a problem of being mindful of which fermentable foods you should eat and which fermentable foods you should avoid.

Simply put, eat an apple instead of toast. Or consider these daily dietary swaps:

- Start your day with high protein and fat, like a eggs and turkey bacon, or a nutrient-packed smoothie instead of whole grain cereal, a muffin, or toast.
- For lunch, opt for a hearty salad with grilled chicken slices in place of a whole grain sandwich.
- As a satisfying snack, carrots and celery sticks paired with hummus offer a satisfying alternative to whole grain crackers, cookies, chips, or any processed snacks.
- Come dinnertime, trade whole wheat pasta or brown rice for spaghetti squash, zucchini noodles, or cauliflower rice, all of which provide fiber and a delightful texture for better colon fermentation.
- Finally, for dessert, you can indulge in sliced fruit or a fruit medley instead of a highly-processed anti-nutrient-riddled dessert. The natural sweetness of these fruits pairs beautifully with their soluble fiber content, creating a gut-friendly treat that satisfies your sweet tooth. Dark chocolate is a good occasional replacement as well!

These simple yet impactful dietary changes allow you to prioritize fermentable foods like fruits and vegetables, contributing to healthy digestion, while avoiding highly fermentable whole grains that might intensify gut inflammation. This can easily be done by replacing high-processed packaged foods with fruits and veggies. Highly processed packaged foods tend to stimulate increased hunger, leading to overeating and chronic colonic fermentation. On the other hand, fruits and vegetables can satisfy your hunger, promoting a feeling of fullness, and support healthy, regular colon fermentation.

Simply put, packaged and processed foods will make you want to eat more (and therefore cause you to eat more) - causing bad fermentation in the colon. Whereas fruits and veggies will satiate your appetite (make you feel full) and cause good fermentation in the colon.

FERMENTABLE FOOD INDEX

LOW

HIGH

Lowest Fermentable Foods:

1. Blueberries
2. Strawberries
3. Grapes
4. Zucchini
5. Carrots
6. Spinach
7. Bell peppers
8. Cucumbers
9. Quinoa
10. Oats
11. Rice
12. Eggs

Highest Fermentable Foods:

1. Onion
2. Garlic
3. Wheat
4. Avocado
5. Artificial sweeteners
6. Apples
7. Pears
8. Watermelon
9. Rye
10. Milk
11. Yogurt
12. Legumes like beans and lentils

Now, does this mean that you shouldn't eat apples or avocados because they are highly fermentable? Not at all. In fact, so long a food has enough of the *right type of fiber*, its high fermentability could be a good thing. For now, focus more on low fermentable foods while still trying to get 20-40g of soluble fiber per day.

SOLUBLE VS **INSOLUBLE** FIBER FOOD LIST

SOLUBLE FIBER	INSOLUBLE FIBER
1. Apples	1. Whole Wheat
2. Citrus Fruits	2. Brown Rice
3. Berries	3. Quinoa
4. Carrots	4. Wheat Bran
5. Chia Seeds	5. Cabbage
6. Sweet Potatoes	6. Broccoli
7. Psyllium Husk	7. Cauliflower
8. Bananas	8. Green Leafy Vegetables (e.g., kale, spinach)
9. Pears	9. Celery
10. Brussels Sprouts	10. Cucumbers

Now, does this mean that you shouldn't eat broccoli, celery, cucumbers, or cabbage because they are dense with insoluble fiber? Not at all, so long your diet has enough of the *right type of fiber (soluble)*. For now, focus more on soluble fiber foods while still trying to get 20-40g per day.

It's worth noting that the fermentability of certain foods can vary depending on individual gut health and tolerance. It's important to listen to your body (or seek advice from a professional when needed) and make dietary choices that work best for your specific needs and digestive comfort.

Non-fermentable Foods

Just as fruits and vegetables are often hailed as the heroes of fermentable foods, it's equally important to shed light on the significance of non-fermentable foods - such as lean proteins and non-starchy vegetables.

While fermentable foods have their place in our diets, it's essential to recognize that they can sometimes trigger excessive consumption. The appeal of their flavors and textures might inadvertently lead to overeating and prolonged colonic fermentation, which, in turn, exacerbates inflammation. On the contrary, non-fermentable foods stand out as the steady and reliable components of a well-rounded diet. They excel in satiating hunger (leaving a lasting sense of fullness) and give your colon a break from having to constantly ferment.

What makes non-fermentable foods particularly appealing is their profile: low in carbohydrates and minimal impact on blood sugar levels. This characteristic not only ensures stable and sustained energy levels but also helps to keep inflammation at bay. In essence, non-fermentable foods provide a strong foundation for overall health by offering essential nutrients while reducing the risk of gut inflammation or digestive discomfort.

While both fermentable and non-fermentable foods have their place on our plates, the importance of making mindful choices cannot be overstated. This is especially critical when it comes to animal produce. There's a world of difference between grain-fed beef and its grass-fed counterpart, just as there is between farm-raised eggs and pasture-raised ones, or even wild caught fish versus farm raised fish. The quality of these food sources can significantly impact the nutritional value they provide and their influence on your overall health.

When you drink alcohol, your body has to work harder to break it down. This leaves less energy for other important processes, such as using carbohydrates, fats, and proteins for energy. This can lead to weight gain, fatigue, impaired coordination, and those dreadful hangovers.

So, why does the body exert extra effort to break down alcohol? Initially, alcohol metabolism takes precedence over other metabolic activities in the liver. The body does this because alcohol is highly toxic, and the liver's top priority is to quickly process and eliminate it. As a result, the normal processing of nutrients from carbs, fats, and proteins temporarily takes a backseat. This metabolic process involves the detoxification of a harmful substance known as acetaldehyde (as mentioned before) which demands additional energy resources from the body, and thus causing the body to work harder.

The destructive impact of alcohol on the gut lining adds another layer to the complexity of its effects on the body. While alcohol metabolism takes precedence in the liver due to its toxicity, the repercussions extend beyond the liver itself. Alcohol tastes bitter, and in its more potent forms it clearly burns your throat when you drink it, right? Imagine what that is doing to your digestive lining. Chronic alcohol consumption can lead to the breakdown of the gut barrier, known as "leaky gut" (as mentioned before), which allows harmful toxins and bacteria to enter the bloodstream. This triggers an immune response and thus inflammation, compounding the overall strain on the body.

Additionally, alcohol is calorie-dense, providing approximately 7 calories per gram, but it lacks essential nutrients like vitamins and minerals. Compare this to carbs and proteins at 4 calories per gram, the only difference being the source of calories from the carbs and proteins being full of essential nutrients and vitamins. So another way to decrease your calorie intake is to decrease your alcohol intake which will also decrease inflammation. As your body metabolizes alcohol, it expends energy that could otherwise be used for processing actual vital nutrients.

The intoxicating consequences of alcohol (like hangovers) are a testament to the intricate and energy-intensive nature of alcohol metabolism. In essence, your body's "hard work" in breaking down alcohol deprioritizes vital nutrient metabolism, toxifies the liver, destroys gut lining, and chronically inflames the body.

As claimed, the consumption of alcohol requires its transformation of ethanol to acetaldehyde, which is associated with the not-so-pleasant experiences of alcohol intoxication, namely hangovers and inflammation. Acetaldehyde is a toxic compound that contributes to hangovers, nausea, and vomiting. It is also a carcinogen, which means that it can cause cancer. The body tries to get rid of acetaldehyde as quickly as possible, but if you drink too much alcohol, the body cannot keep up and acetaldehyde levels compound. This is what causes the lasting head-pounding effects of a hangover.

It is important to note that excessive alcohol consumption can lead to specific conditions such as alcoholic hepatitis, pancreatitis, and fatty liver disease. With that said, alcohol consumption has peripheral implications on weight gain, metabolism issues, heart problems, and more. Individuals with preexisting inflammatory conditions may find their symptoms exacerbated when alcohol triggers inflammation in their bodies. This is a concern that many of my clients have encountered in the past. Throughout the week, they would maintain a healthy diet and engage in regular exercise. However, on the weekends, they would indulge in excessive drinking to unwind. While this was not an issue for some, those with specific intolerances would experience a significant setback in their health and wellness due to the detrimental effects of the alcohol.

To use a specific example, I had a client who would eat perfect all work week, Monday through Friday. He would track his macronutrient numbers, successfully meet those macronutrient numbers, stayed hydrated, followed the workout program that I customized for him to a tee, and did everything that was asked of him.

Yet, when Saturday and Sunday came (especially during football season), he would drink a few shots and some beer. He never told me exactly how much he drank, but he said he would never get 'blasted' and would rarely get hangovers. He still got healthier from when we first started, no doubt, and had lost nearly 50 pounds. But once he got to a certain "healthier" he plateaued, and his progress started to stagnate. He looked better and felt better, but he wanted to look even better and feel even better. It wasn't until we went on an 8 week "no alcohol" detox that he began to climb out of that stagnation. After 8 weeks of no alcohol, he started looking even better and feeling even better.

I've had other clients who were able to balance weekly alcohol consumption and still maintain progress in their fitness journey, although those clients would've looked and felt even better if they'd cut out the alcohol entirely. Whether you choose to consume alcohol or not, no matter how regular, it is crucial for individuals with preexisting inflammatory conditions to be aware of the potential risks associated with alcohol consumption and make informed decisions accordingly. And without you having to take a comprehensive test to determine your preexisting inflammatory conditions, you can ensure the decreasing of inflammation by limiting your alcohol consumption altogether.

Knowing about the complex relationship between alcohol, energy metabolism, and inflammation empowers us to make informed decisions about alcohol consumption. While infrequent alcohol intake may not pose significant issues, frequent or excessive alcohol consumption disrupts the body's preferred energy sources and leads to a variety of health problems. So long you accept alcohol as a literal poison that is toxic to your body, then hey, drink responsibly

For individuals dealing with gut inflammation, it is essential to prioritize non-fermentable foods over fermentable ones. This approach helps reduce the risk of further aggravating gut inflammation and supports digestive health. As Americans, we could all benefit from decreasing the amount of fermentable foods that we eat, even though there is significant benefit to certain fermentable foods. The primary fermentable foods that we should prioritize are soluble fibers..

Ultimately, dietary choices should still be based on unique preferences, tolerances, and individual goals. Consulting with a healthcare professional can provide personalized guidance to create a balanced meal plan that minimizes gut inflammation and maximizes the benefits of certain fermentable and non-fermentable options for gut health and weight management.

Considering the prevalence of gut inflammation among many Americans, understanding the fermentability of foods becomes crucial for promoting proper digestive health and weight management. While fermentable foods can offer benefits such as lower energy density and satiety (feeling full), they may exacerbate gut inflammation for individuals with preexisting digestive issues. Prioritizing healthier fermentable foods (namely soluble fibers) and non-fermentable foods (such as lean proteins and non-starchy vegetables) becomes essential in managing gut inflammation for the average American. Through educating ourselves, we can begin making informed choices in generally reducing an overly-fermented diet. It is through making informed nutritional decisions where we can work towards relieving our gut inflammation, optimizing digestion, and achieving the success of becoming a healthier and happier version of ourselves.

In Chapter 6, we will discuss specific digestive inflammatory compounds known as "anti-nutrients" named lectins, oxalates, phytates, and industrialized seed oils. These anti-nutrients interrupt our body's ability to absorb nutrients, destroy our gut lining, and so much more. Similar to the effects of alcohol and excess sugar, we will discover how anti-nutrients contain compounds that erode at our gut lining. Reference back to the analogy of our digestive system being like a plumbing system. Envision your digestive system as a plumbing network where your mouth serves as your home's toilet, and your anus acts as the city's sewage system. Just as you'd only flush materials down your home's toilet that wouldn't obstruct the plumbing or harm its pipe-lining, your gut must maintain the integrity of its plumbing to prevent chronic inflammation.

What would happen if you flushed a bunch of nails down your toilet? That's what consuming anti-nutrients is like. While a single nail or two may not inflict considerable damage, the cumulative effect of flushing more nails over time would lead to the gradual degradation of the plumbing system's structural integrity. Once the protective lining of the plumbing system is compromised, it may result in the seepage of sewage into the very foundation of your house - a situation best preempted and prevented.

Chapter 6

Exploring Anti-Nutrients: Lectins, Oxalates, Phytates, and Industrialized Seed Oils

Whole foods are key - except whole grains.

Since the dawn of agriculture, nearly every major civilization has woven legumes (such as lentils, peas, beans, soy, chickpeas, peanuts) and grains into the fabric of their diet. From barley and lentils in one part of the world to the pairing of corn or rice with beans in another. These staples have been part of the human diet for centuries. However, the way in which they were prepared and consumed, as well as the balance between how much was consumed, dignified the overall nutritious harmony of ancient diets.

It is between the nuanced interplay between quantity and quality of food where nutritional richness and healthy habits are found. The grains and foods we eat are not the grains and foods that our ancestors ate, and this concept holds the key to understanding why certain foods did not manifest the same toxic diseases for our ancestors as they do for us.

The primary reason why so many modern humans are unhealthy is due to gluttony. Even if you do not overeat and aren't obese, the odds of you still consuming certain anti-nutrients in gluttonous quantities is very likely (due to most foods being so processed). And this isn't necessarily your fault - or wasn't your fault at least. Now and going forward, however, you have no choice but to take fault for the overconsumption of certain anti-nutrients. Plus, once you realize what anti-nutrients are doing to your body, you'll mindfully limit their overconsumption anyway.

There are plenty of anti-nutrients to be weary of, but most aren't as pesky or prevalent as a group of natural compounds known as lectins, oxalates, and phytates. Though these compounds are essential in various plant-based foods, they also serve as formidable defensive compounds against plant predators. Simply put, plants contain certain toxic compounds that are hardwired into their biology to act as defensive deterrents to dissuade animals from eating them. This is why understanding their potential impact on human health is so important, as excessive consumption of these compounds will pose specific challenges.

Additionally, we will discuss the anti-nutrient make-up of industrialized seed oils and how their processing methods, which often involve high-pressure extraction, bleaching, and toxic chemical treatments, harm your health.

In this chapter, we will discuss which foods contain these compounds, which foods to avoid, and the intricate relationship between different anti-nutrients and your body.

One aspect that distinguishes anti-nutrients like lectins, oxalates, and phytates from normal dietary nutrients is their resistance to breakdown by human digestive enzymes. This means that when we consume foods containing lectins or any other anti-nutrients, these compounds can remain intact as they pass through our digestive tract. And as they pass through the digestive tract undigested, they affect the digestive lining like a flushed nail would affect a plumbing's lining. However, it's important to note that not all anti-nutrients are created equal, and their potential effects can vary depending on the type of anti-nutrient, the amount consumed, and individual tolerance.

Lectins

Lectins are a type of protein found in many plant foods, including grains, legumes, and certain fruits and vegetables.
In plants, lectins act as a defense mechanism, deterring predators such as insects and animals from consuming them. These compounds bind to specific molecules and disrupt cellular function - causing harm to the predator. When ingested by humans, lectins interact with the lining of the digestive tract like a flushed nail would interact with a plumbing's pipe-lining. Sure, a few nails here and there won't do much harm, but if you flush enough nails (or eat enough anti-nutrients) then you'll begin to compromise your plumbing's lining.

It's important to note that the extent of lectin-related health concerns (like many, if-not-all, health concerns) varies among individuals, as everyone's tolerance and sensitivity to compounds can differ (whether that's lectins, oxalates, phytates, gluten, lactose, you name it). This is known as genetic heterogeneity which simply means we are all uniquely different and genetically respond differently to foods to varying degrees.

It's worth emphasizing that the potential negative effects of lectin-ladened foods (again, like most compounds) are often associated with how the food is prepared and how much of the food is consumed. When it comes to lectins, the emphasis lies in raw or undercooked foods. In their unprocessed state, lectin-dense foods retain their lectin content, whereas cooking and preparing them properly severely diminished the lectin content. Traditional methods such as cooking, soaking, and fermenting have long been recognized as essential methods in reducing anti-nutrient content and enhancing the safety and digestibility of these foods.

For instance, let's consider beans. When consumed in their raw or undercooked state, they contain elevated lectin levels which your body begins to respond negatively towards - usually resulting in chronic nausea and vomiting. Throughout human history, our ancestors intuitively harnessed the power of certain cooking methods to transform beans into a safer and more nutritious dietary staple. Pressure cooking beans, for example, is crucial in order to remove their toxic lectin content, whereas slow cooking them will not. Proper cooking significantly reduces lectin levels, making foods like beans not only more palatable but also more vital.

Another class example is our ancestors' profound understanding of rice and wheat transformation. This is most evident by the preference for white rice over brown rice, originating from a clever strategy to remove lectins and anti-nutrients. In this culinary evolution, the outer hull, rich in lectins and anti-nutrients, was meticulously stripped away to create the familiar white rice. They first harvested the mature rice grains and then dried them in the sun to reduce moisture. The next crucial step involved dehulling, which expertly removed the tough outer hull from each rice kernel through abrasion (usually the grinding between two stones). The subsequent milling stage further refines the rice by eliminating the bran layer and germ, where much of the lectins and anti-nutrients were concentrated. The final result was white rice, which, although lower in some nutrients, became a safer and more digestible dietary staple, reflecting centuries of culinary wisdom.

Similarly, in the case of wheat, unless a similar dehulling process is employed, the resulting flour remains coarse, retaining the bran layer rich in lectins and anti-nutrients. The consequence is a dense, whole wheat flour that, like brown rice, maintains the presence of these undesired compounds. This parallel can be drawn with the process of refining whole grain "brown" rice to create white rice, where the removal of the toxic outer hull ensures a safer and more digestible final product. While it's true that white rice and white bread are less nutritionally dense compared to their whole grain counterparts, it's essential to consider the trade-off between nutritional density and the presence of potentially harmful compounds. I do not recommend eating white bread, so a simple solution is if you're going to eat bread, you need to make sure it is at least *gluten free,* as gluten is considered a type of lectin. Whole grain products, including brown rice and whole wheat bread, indeed contain more vitamins, minerals, and dietary fiber (although the fiber from grains is primarily *insoluble fiber*). However, they also tend to be denser in toxic compounds like lectins and other anti-nutrients.

The question then becomes whether the additional nutrients found in whole grains compensate for the potential drawbacks. In many cases, people can obtain these essential nutrients from other dietary sources, allowing them to opt for white rice or gluten free options while minimizing their exposure to excess lectins and other anti-nutrients. Ultimately, the choice between whole grains and refined grains should be guided by individual dietary needs, preferences, and individual health considerations.

Oxalates

Oxalates, also known as oxalic acid, are naturally occurring compounds found in various plant-based foods, particularly in leafy greens, certain vegetables, and fruits. In plants, oxalates serve as a protective mechanism against herbivores and predators. These compounds have a unique ability to bind with calcium, forming insoluble crystals called calcium oxalate, which can lead to kidney stones.

Much like lectins, the impact of oxalates on human health can vary from person to person due to genetic heterogeneity. While some individuals may tolerate oxalates well, others might experience adverse effects when ingesting foods with high oxalate content. It's important to be aware of oxalate-rich foods and consider moderation in consumption to minimize potential health risks. Cooking, boiling, baking, or roasting can also help reduce oxalate levels in foods, making them more suitable for those with heightened sensitivity to these compounds. For example, kale and spinach are high in oxalates and therefore should not be eaten raw, rather they should be boiled or blanched. After cooking, the oxalic acid will be concentrated in the water and can then be discarded.

Phytates

Phytates, also known as phytic acid, are prevalent in whole grain products, legumes, nuts, and seeds, and they have a unique role in both health and nutrition. On one hand, phytates are recognized for their antioxidant properties and certain potential health benefits. However, they are also considered anti-nutrients due to their mineral-binding properties, which can interfere with the absorption of essential minerals like calcium, iron, and zinc. This aspect has raised concerns about potential mineral deficiencies, particularly for those who consume a diet rich in phytic acid. So, like the trade-off with whole grains that offer more vitamins and minerals but are more dense in compounds like lectins and phytic acid, the question arises: do the additional nutrients found in anti-nutrient—rich foods compensate for their potential drawbacks? The answer, as with whole grains, often depends on individual dietary needs and preferences. Many essential nutrients found in lectin-rich, oxalic acid-rich, and phytic acid-rich foods can also be obtained from alternative dietary sources. Simply put, you don't have to eat whole grains, legumes/beans, oats, or corn to get the good nutrients that they have to offer. In fact, in many cases it's not worth eating these foods and you can find their "good nutrients" elsewhere without risking the drawbacks of their anti-nutrients.

Industrialized Seed Oils

It's not as though the fatty acids or "oils" in plants and seeds are inherently bad, it's when they are super heated and industrially processed where they begin to become oxidized, rancid, and toxic for the body.

The Industrial Revolution marked a transformative era characterized by technological advancements and the rise of steel machinery. These machines, essential to the world's rapid industrialization, required effective lubrication to maintain smooth operations. Traditionally, whale fat served as a staple lubricant and played a critical role in illuminating lamps and powering machinery. Additionally, oils such as olive oil, which had been used since ancient Egyptian times for moving large objects, were heavily relied upon.

However, the extensive utilization of whale blubber for various applications, including candle/soap production, oils for lamps, and lubrication, led to a growing scarcity of this resource. The hunting of whales to near extinction and their subsequent depletion of providing blubber for oil prompted a search for more accessible, cost-effective alternatives to meet the increasing demand for industrial soaps, candles, lamps, and lubricants.

The 1800s witnessed the flourishing rise of the cotton industry, largely due to the invention of the cotton gin. This innovation streamlined cotton processing, being able to sift cotton seeds from cotton lint, resulting in a significant boost in overall production.

However, this surge in cotton output posed a major predicament for cotton producers: the accumulation of inedible and useless cottonseeds. Before the development of industrial applications for cotton seeds, farmers had limited options for surplus seeds. They could use some for planting in the following year's crop, but there was usually a surplus that had no immediate use. These excess seeds were often discarded or left to accumulate as waste, posing a disposal challenge for cotton producers.

During this critical juncture, two entrepreneurs, candle-maker William Procter and soap-maker James Gamble, recognized a unique opportunity to reduce production costs for their respective industries. Leveraging emerging technology, like a pioneering process known as "hydrogenation", Procter and Gamble were able to transform liquid cottonseed oil into a solid, creamy, butter-like fat. They patented two techniques for hydrogenating cottonseed oil. While their original purpose was to fully solidify the oils for soap production, these methods also enabled the oil to stay in a solid state at typical storage temperatures, making it suitable for the food industry.

In 1911, the creation of industrialized seed oils was introduced to the public under the name "Crisco" and was marketed as a healthier and more American alternative to traditional sources of dietary fat, such as butter, lard, and tallow. This marked a pivotal moment in American nutrition history, where seed oils began their ascent to dominance. Before the widespread use of such seed oils, our ancestors relied on natural fats like butter, tallow, lard, olive oil, and coconut oil for various cooking and dietary purposes for thousands of years.

Procter and Gamble's product, Crisco, rapidly gained popularity and international success by 1921. Their influence extended to the financing of health organizations, notably the American Heart Association.

In 1948, the American Heart Association received financial support from Procter and Gamble, setting the stage for a significant shift in dietary recommendations and public perception of fats and oils.

In 1955, a significant turning point occurred when President Eisenhower suffered a "heart attack" that brought national awareness to the severity of what would later be known as "cardiovascular disease." This event prompted a national outcry for measures to prevent heart disease. Just six years later, in 1961, the American Heart Association endorsed and funded the Ancel Keys "Diet-Heart Hypothesis," which suggested that saturated fats from sources like butter, tallow, lard, olive oil, and coconut oil were the primary contributors to heart attacks, while polyunsaturated fats derived from seed oils were touted as the solution to preventing unhealthy cardiovascular conditions. This marked a significant shift in the realm of nutrition and cardiovascular health, especially considering that heart attacks and heart disease had been relatively foreign and uncommon in American society until the mid-1900s. Consequently, seed oils, once viewed primarily as industrial lubricants, took center stage as the American solution to heart attacks.

This transformation had profound implications as cardiovascular disease began its ascent to becoming the leading global cause of mortality. The shift in dietary preferences from traditional saturated fats to the promotion of seed oils had far-reaching consequences for global health.

Again, it's not as though the polyunsaturated fatty acids or "oils" in plants and seeds are inherently bad, it's when they are consumed in excess, super heated, and industrially transformed where they begin to become oxidized, rancid, and toxic for the body.

The production process of these oils is a multi-step procedure that begins with the extraction of oil from seeds. Let's look at the industrial production of canola oil, to illustrate.

The seeds undergo high-pressure pressing, effectively converting the seeds into a cake/gum-like substance. This gummy cake must then be degummed and turned into a liquid, which introduces the use of a toxic compound called hexane as a dissolving solvent (hexane is a neurotoxin that can leave its traces within the oil). This initial process already sets the stage for future health risks. The hexane-ladened oil then undergoes further cleaning, which includes exposing it to temperatures exceeding 400 degrees Fahrenheit. This high-temperature processing leads to the degradation of the seed's natural nutritious value - causing the oil to spoil and smell rancid.

But we're still not done. Now you've got a stinky, yet "edible", distilled seed oil that is opaque and unappealing. In order to make this degraded, yet "edible", seed oil more commercially attractive, the oil is further refined with sodium hydroxide (a known carcinogen, meaning cancer-causing compound) in order to deodorize the rancid smell, and is then literally bleached to make the oil more clear. The goal of these processing steps is to produce clear, odorless, and flavorless oils that have a longer shelf life and are suitable for various culinary and industrial applications.

Just think about that for a second.

To make things worse, seed oils are pervasive in nearly all packaged foods due to their cost-effectiveness, ability to extend shelf life, enhance texture and palatability, serve as flavor carriers, and withstand high-temperature cooking. Their stability prevents products from spoiling rapidly, an essential factor in the world of packaged goods.

Additionally, they contribute to the creamy or satisfying feel in various foods, making them more appealing to consumers. Their high smoke points are crucial for frying and cooking at high temperatures, which is common in the preparation of many packaged items. Moreover, seed oils play a role in preserving the quality and taste of food products over time - making them taste good by not spoiling for a long time. However, excessive use of seed oils in the food industry can lead to an unhealthy imbalance of omega-6 fatty acids in the diet, making it important for consumers to be mindful of the types and quantities of fats and oils in their packaged foods to maintain a balanced and nutritious diet.

That is truly the worst part about industrialized seed oils; their dense omega-6 fatty acid content, namely arachidonic acid in excess. I am sure you are familiar with omega-3 fatty acids, like from fish oils, and if you're not, then simply understand this: omega-3 fatty acids contain crucial anti-inflammatory fatty compounds known as APA, DHA and EPA, and omega-6 fatty acids contain a specific inflammatory compound known as arachidonic acid. To put it in perspective, the human brain is made up of nearly 2/3 of fat, and the vast majority of that fat is made up of DHA. Without boring you with what this means and what this potentially implicates, just know that dolphins, orcas, and humans are all incredibly smart because of the DHA content in our ancestors' diets. DHA, in more recent studies, has proven to literally grow the brain, and particularly grow the hippocampus (memory center of the brain), which further substantiates the importance of omega-3s - namely DHA.

While both omega-6 and omega-3 fatty acids are essential for our health, the modern American diet has disrupted the delicate balance by significantly tilting it towards omega-6s. It's easiest to think of omega-3's as anti-inflammatory and omega-6's as pro-inflammatory.

The ideal ratio for an omega-3 to omega-6 distribution would be 1:1 to 1:3. The average American maintains an omega-3 to omega-6 ratio of 1:20 at minimum,[1] and most health experts would agree it could be much, much higher than that. This skewed ratio can have dire consequences as omega-6 fatty acids, when excessively consumed, promote inflammation.

While natural sources of omega-6 fatty acids are present in whole foods like nuts and seeds, their unrestricted overconsumption through the widespread use of these processed oils is where the peril truly lies.

The odyssey of industrialized seed oils, as revealed through the production of cottonseed oil and canola oil, is a stark illustration of the intricate relationship between these oils and human health.

I am strongly recommending you either fully remove or severely limit your intake of seed oils. I am not, however, telling you to completely remove whole grains, beans, oats, or corn from your diet. I am simply exposing the overall effects that these foods could cause in impacting your health. Reference back to the introductory chapter where I express the importance of limiting your dietary degeneracy.

Remember, eating healthy is not about deprivation. It's about making sustainable choices that will nourish your body and mind. And since everybody's body is different, we must take into account the way in which certain foods and compounds may affect each one of our unique physiologies. I always tell my clients that a healthy diet deserves dessert every night, and to think of healthy eating as a percentage distribution - aiming for a minimum of 80% clean and allowing for 20% flexibility for indulgence. When you consistently prioritize clean eating, you 'earn the right' to enjoy occasional rewards within that 20%. Now, defining what that dessert looks like and qualifying it within that 20% is a separate conversation altogether.
With that said, so long you can compartmentalize the consumption of anti-nutrients within a 20% 'earned' indulgence window, I don't see a problem enjoying the occasional donut or candy bar. The key word there would be *occasional,* and not surpassing that 20% window.

In unveiling the truth about lectins, oxalates, and phytates, we gain a deeper insight to their roles as protective compounds in plants and their implications on human health. Armed with this knowledge, we can make informed choices about how we either incorporate or avoid these foods in our diets, striking a balance between their potential benefits and their toxic potential. Not only this, we now have a better comprehensive understanding of why industrialized seed oils are so bad and how they inadvertently began decaying American health in response to convenience and profit.

Understanding the nuances of what we consume allows us to make informed decisions about how we nourish our bodies.

Chapter 7 will build on this knowledge as we explore the significance of mindful eating habits. We'll discuss how to avoid anti-nutrients and harmful seed oils and replace them with healthier alternatives, which is essential for fostering a healthier, more conscious approach to fueling our bodies.

Chapter 7

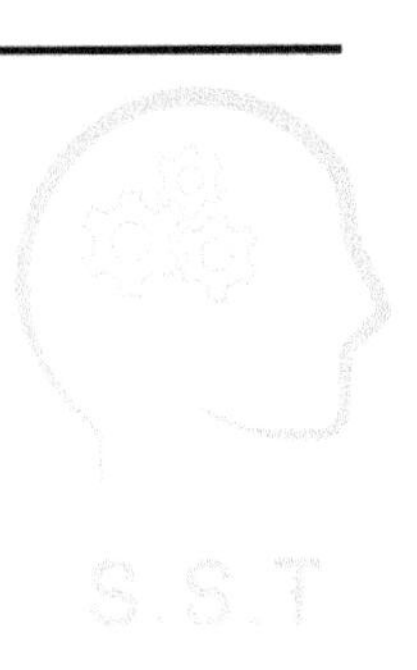

Smart Snacking and Mindful Eating Habits

In today's fast-paced world, where it's easy to eat on the go or in front of screens without paying attention to what we're eating, practicing mindful eating habits can help us cultivate a healthier relationship with food.

Mindful eating involves being fully engaged with our eating experience, using all of our senses to savor the flavors, textures, and aromas of our food while being aware of our body's hunger and fullness cues. When we combine the principles of mindful eating with smart snacking, we can make conscious choices that promote both nourishment and enjoyment.

Smart snacking is important for several reasons. First, snacks can provide an energy boost throughout the day, helping us overcome afternoon slumps and maintain productivity. They allow us to incorporate additional nutrients into our diet, ensuring we meet our nutritional needs. Smart snacking can also help us control our calorie intake, supporting weight management and preventing overeating during meals.

When it comes to nutritious and satisfying snack ideas, there are numerous options available. Fresh or dried fruits, sliced vegetables with dips, smoothies, a handful of mixed nuts or seeds - the options are endless. Foods like Greek yogurt offers a protein-rich and customizable snack with flexible toppings.

Avoiding unhealthy snacks and mindless eating requires some planning and awareness. And, sadly, the majority of food in any given food mart is likely unhealthy. When you walk into any mainline grocery store, you can generally assume that everything packaged and shelved is highly processed and refined (reference last chapter, as seed oils are inside nearly all the packaged food that we buy). With that said, it is important to read the back of ingredient labels and qualify whether or not the ingredients include any seed oils - which most, if not all, will contain one or two+ different seed oils, namely soybean.

To make reading ingredient lists or qualifying a packaged food's toxic potential easier, opt for shopping around the perimeter of the grocery store and start buying less packaged/processed foods. While seed oils are commonly used in many packaged and processed foods to extend shelf life, frozen foods are preserved through the freezing process itself, which inhibits the growth of microorganisms that cause food to spoil. Some frozen foods, like frozen fruits and vegetables, are typically free from added oils, while others, like frozen fried products, may have some form of oil or fat for flavor or texture. When choosing frozen foods, it's essential to read the ingredient labels to understand what has been added to them.

Though it may be challenging for the average American to completely eliminate seed oils from their diet, everyone can take steps to address the overconsumption of conveniently delicious seed-oil-products. Choose more nutritious alternatives, like apples instead of candy bars, or grapes in place of cookies. Substitute chips with carrots, and swap sandwiches for salads. I personally am an avid lover of chocolate, so I opt for dark chocolate over commercial chocolate to fulfill my coco-cravings. If you find the taste of dark chocolate alone a bit strong, you can complement it by pairing it with fruits such as strawberries, berries, or bananas. You can also enhance the experience by dipping covered almonds or your preferred healthy alternative into melted dark chocolate. Planning and preparing wholesome snacks in advance empowers us to resist the lure of less healthy options when hunger strikes.

When it comes to mindful eating habits, being mindful of portion sizes helps us avoid excessive calorie intake, while practicing mindful eating encourages us to savor each bite and enjoy the sensory experience of our snacks. To engage in mindful eating, take the time to slow down and savor each bite. Pay attention to the taste, texture, and smell of your food. Put down your utensils between bites and chew your food thoroughly before swallowing. Engage with the colors and aromas that arise with each mouthful, truly experiencing the pleasure of eating.

Listening to your body's signals of hunger and fullness is also crucial. Before eating, check in with yourself to assess your level of hunger. Eat until you are satisfied, not overly full, and pause during the meal to gauge your fullness level. By tuning into these cues, you can honor your body's needs and prevent overeating.

Creating a calm and quiet eating environment is another aspect of mindful eating. Minimize distractions such as screens, phones, or other disturbances. Instead, focus solely on the act of eating and the enjoyment of your meal. Use this time to practice gratitude for the nourishment provided by the food on your plate. How grateful would your ancestors be for the immediacy and surplus of food that you currently have at your disposal?

Planning ahead, being mindful of portion sizes, practicing mindfulness, and avoiding distractions can all contribute to a healthier snacking experience. With these strategies in place, we can embrace smart snacking as a sustainable part of our healthy lifestyle, supporting energy levels, satisfaction, and our personal health goals.

Another key aspect to mindful eating is being able to recognize emotional triggers that may lead to unhealthy eating patterns. This deserves its own book altogether, but for now try to understand that mindless eating or eating because we're bored is an easy way to feel good. Highly processed foods often contain both sugar and seed oils, making them highly palatable and appealing to our taste buds. These ingredients are used by the food industry to create products that are not only tasty but also addictive. Sugar provides a sweet and pleasurable taste, while seed oils can enhance the mouthfeel and texture of these foods, making them more appealing.

The connection between highly processed foods and mindless eating, driven by emotional triggers or boredom, is deeply rooted in the brain's reward system. When we consume these foods, they trigger the release of dopamine in the brain, creating a pleasurable sensation. Dopamine is a neurotransmitter associated with the brain's reward center and is often referred to as the "feel-good" chemical. This neurological response can lead to emotional eating, where we seek comfort or distraction from negative emotions by indulging in such foods.

The same brain regions associated with drug addiction are involved in this process, contributing to the concept that these highly processed foods can be seen as providing "free dopamine hits" and offering a form of "free drug hits." Over time, this can lead to unhealthy eating patterns and, in some cases, even addiction-like behaviors towards unhealthy foods.

Recognizing and addressing emotional triggers and mindless eating is essential for promoting mindful eating habits. This involves developing an awareness of the emotional and psychological factors that influence our food choices and finding healthier ways to cope with these emotions. By doing so, we can regain control over our eating habits and make more conscious and healthful food choices. Engaging in stress-reducing activities, journaling, or seeking support from loved ones or a professional can help address emotional eating and develop a healthier relationship with food. Seeking help from a professional to overcome or further diagnose solution paths for an eating disorder is important, but most people can remedy this addiction-like compulsion by replacing bad foods with good foods, and learning to enjoy the healthier options. Over time, your brain will be as appreciative to the juicy sweetness of an apple as it does for the sweetness of chocolate chip cookies. Does that mean that chocolate chip cookies aren't more palatable and, in a way, more delicious? Probably not for the majority of us. But you can train your brain to crave an apple in the same way it craves a sugary chocolate chip cookie.

Be mindful of external influences, such as food marketing and societal pressures. Stay true to your own needs and preferences, and listen to your body's cues when making food choices. Trust yourself to make decisions that align with your healthy-living standards. We will discuss this more in depth in the next chapter.

Through integrating mindful eating and smart snacking into our daily lives, we can develop a healthier and more conscious relationship with food. Slow down, savor each bite, and truly engage with the present moment. Choose nutrient-dense snacks that nourish your body and practice portion control. Overcome challenges by prioritizing your well-being, addressing emotional triggers, and staying true to yourself. Digest these habits as lifelong sustainable practices so that you can embrace living as your healthiest self.

Chapter 8

Savoring Social Situations and Dining Out

Humans are inherently social creatures, and our connections with others play a vital role in our health. Though humans do not socialize to the same capacity that our ancestors once did, we still require quality time with the people that we love. Whether it's sharing a meal with loved ones, meeting friends for a night out, or attending social events, our social interactions provide us with a sense of belonging, joy, and fulfillment. However, when it comes to sustaining a healthy nutrition plan, navigating social situations and dining out can pose challenges. In this chapter, we will explore practical strategies and tips for making healthier choices while still savoring social situations and dining out.

Dining out and navigating social situations can be a double-edged sword. On one hand, it's an opportunity to let loose and savor delicious food, explore new cuisines, and bond with others. On the other hand, it can present temptations, unhealthy options, and a departure from our regular routine. When it comes to dining out, planning ahead is a secret weapon. Take advantage of the opportunity to review the menu online before you head out. By doing so, you can identify healthier options and decide what you will order in advance. This simple step helps you avoid impulsive and less healthy choices influenced by enticing menu descriptions or the preferences of your dining companions. When browsing the menu, prioritize dishes that emphasize lean proteins, an adequate amount of vegetables, and try to avoid overly-fried food. Opt for grilled, baked, or steamed preparations rather than fried or breaded options.

Another crucial aspect of dining out is within a discipline that we've already hammered down: portion control. It's no secret that restaurant servings (especially in America) tend to be larger than what we truly need. To avoid overeating, consider sharing an entrée with a dining partner or ask for a take-out container at the beginning of the meal to pack up leftovers. Being mindful of portion sizes helps you maintain a balanced approach and prevents excessive gluttony.

And this gluttonous behavior should be more emphasized when it comes to how much alcohol you drink if you decide to do so. Feel free to reference the entire chapter on alcohol. I don't mean to be a literal buzzkill, but does your buzz need that extra shot or extra beer? Moderation is key, and humans are always going to human. But in order to be healthier than you currently are, you have to be mindful of the karmic debt that gluttonous behavior can bring - especially with regard to alcohol. A simple solution is to mix in a few glasses of water here and there.

Sides and accompaniments will also significantly impact the nutritional value of your meal. Swap high-calorie options like fries or creamy sauces for healthier alternatives such as steamed vegetables or side salads. Don't hesitate to request modifications that align with your dietary preferences, such as the aforementioned substituting breaded items with grilled alternatives. My partner has an autoimmune disorder that requires her to go above and beyond when we dine out - as many restaurants do not accommodate to her autoimmune disorder as well as others. I can assure you that the effort required is minuscule compared to the down-stream effects of not doing some due diligence to align with your dietary preferences or needs. These small adjustments can make a big difference in the overall quality of your dining experience.

Communication is key. Share your commitment to healthy living with your friends and family. I'm not saying to be that family member who solicits unwanted preaching, but for the sake of social circumstances it's crucial to inform your social group on adjustments that you will be making. By informing them of your lifestyle choices, they can take your preferences into consideration when planning meals or gatherings. Believe it or not, this open communication fosters a level of intimacy and support that further nourishes your relationship with those people!

Another approach to social events is to bring a dish yourself. When offering to contribute a healthy and delicious dish, you ensure that there will be at least one option that aligns with your dietary goals. Additionally, sharing your healthy eating choices with others can inspire and encourage them to make healthier choices as well. To such a degree than instead of dining out, you can choose to gather your social circle and dine in. This approach offers control of what/how food is being prepared, and allows you to bring the raving nightlife experience into a more intimate setting. By organizing get-togethers at someone's place, you gain greater control over various elements that dining out might not offer. This change of setting can elevate your social experiences and promote an environment where making healthier choices becomes easier. Explore cooking new healthier dishes with friends or loved ones, and make experimenting with new recipes a part of the fun.

Remember, it's okay to enjoy indulgent foods occasionally. Rather than completely avoiding them, practice moderation and portion control. When dining out with friends or loved ones, allow yourself a small serving of your favorite treat and savor it mindfully. Share a dessert with someone or the group. Focus on the flavors and the social experience, taking pleasure in the moment without overindulging.

To make social gatherings more inclusive of everyone's well-being, shift the focus from being solely centered around food. Plan activities that involve physical movement, such as going for a walk, playing a sport, or exploring fun activities in your city. Diversifying the experience beyond just eating creates an environment that satisfies your natural social craving without having to actually break bread.

Surround yourself with a supportive social network that understands and respects your healthy eating goals. Engage with like-minded individuals who share similar values, provide encouragement, accountability, and make the journey of healthy living more enjoyable and less of a chore.

Chapter 9

Meal Planning and Grocery Shopping Made Easy

Meal planning and grocery shopping are often overlooked steps towards achieving a healthier eating routine. Simply optimizing these two concepts makes staying organized, saving time, and making sustainable food choices much easier. In this chapter, we will break down the benefits of meal planning, provide practical strategies for effective meal planning, and offer tips for smart grocery shopping.

One of the key advantages of meal planning is the time and energy it saves. When we map out our meals in advance, we eliminate the need to make daily decisions about what to cook. With a well-thought-out plan, you can streamline your cooking process, avoid last-minute uncertainties, and reduce stress in the kitchen.

In addition to saving time, meal planning can also help you save money. By creating a comprehensive shopping list based on your meal plan, you will avoid unnecessary impulse purchases and reduce wasteful spending. This mindful approach to grocery shopping ensures that you buy only what you need and maximally utilize your ingredients, leading to long-term financial savings in tandem with healthy eating habits.

Effective meal planning requires dedicated time each week. Find a quiet moment to brainstorm meal ideas, create a menu, and construct a thorough grocery list. Break down what you eat, where you eat, and the cost of each food item.

This deliberate planning process sets the foundation for a successful and stress-free week of meals, exposing and facilitating changes in poor consuming habits.

When grocery shopping, a well-prepared list is crucial. Create a detailed list and stick to your list to avoid impulse purchases of unhealthy snacks or items that contradict your health goals. Focus on fresh foods found in the perimeter of the store—more organic and less processed—while limiting exposure to seed-oil-ladened and packaged foods in the center aisles.

Read food labels and ingredient lists attentively. Choose products with little to no seed oils (preferably none), minimal dyes/additives, and limited added sugars. Choose more organic options (especially with fruit and veggies), high quality protein sources, and foods with recognizable, natural ingredients. Keep a close eye out for those pesky anti-nutrients.

As emphasized earlier, it's crucial to avoid seed oils, such as soybean, corn, canola, cottonseed, safflower, peanut, sunflower, etcetera. Instead, opt for products that contain minimal or no seed oils, and favor healthier cooking alternatives like olive or avocado oil. Secondly, exercise caution when it comes to artificial additives, especially common ones like monosodium glutamate (MSG), high-fructose corn syrup (HFCS), artificial sweeteners like aspartame, saccharin, and sucralose, food colorings such as Red 40 and Yellow 5, and a bevy of artificial flavors. Choose products with natural flavors, fewer or no preservatives. Exploring organic options is crucial when feasible, as organic products are cultivated without synthetic pesticides, GMOs, or synthetic fertilizers and often contain fewer harmful additives. Opt for higher quality protein choices, such as pasture raised poultry, 100% grass-fed meat cuts, wild caught fish, and organic fruits and vegetables. Lastly, embrace products with ingredient lists that feature recognizable and natural ingredients. If you can't pronounce it, you probably should exercise caution when consuming. My general rule of thumb is "*the more ingredients the worse, and the simpler the ingredients the better.*"

Cooking in batches is a game-changer for busy individuals, offering a multitude of benefits. Preparing larger quantities of dishes or ingredients ensures readily available meals throughout the week. This approach streamlines your cooking process, promotes efficient ingredient usage, and satiates the oh-so-necessary fulfillment of convenience.

Batch cooking or "meal prepping" allows you to stockpile pre-prepared components that can be easily incorporated into various meals. Cook a large batch of 100% grass fed beef, white rice, and steamed broccoli and refrigerate or freeze them in portioned containers for quick and nutritious meals. Prepare proteins like grilled chicken breast, lean beef/turkey/bison, et, just find protein sources that you enjoy and can eat pre-prepped. Also, soups and stews, when cooked in larger quantities, provide nourishing meals that can be stored for later consumption. Choose a specific day when you can plan your meals, chop vegetables, marinate proteins, and cook larger batches. I use to do this twice a week, where I would cook a large batch of meals on Sunday evening for Monday, Tuesday, and Wednesday and then I would cook another big batch on Wednesday night for Thursday, Friday, and Saturday. Then on Sunday, I would give myself the freedom to dine out with something healthy, like a steak dinner at a restaurant, then batch cook again that night to restart the routine. This investment of a few hours in advance pays off significantly during busy weekdays, saving you time and reducing stress in the kitchen. As you explore batch cooking, be sure to experiment with flavors and ingredient combinations to add variety and excitement to your meals. The convenience, healthier eating conditions, and enjoyment of the cooking experience make meal prepping a worthwhile strategy for busy individuals seeking efficient and nutritious on-the-go meal solutions.

Meal planning empowers you to make healthier food choices. Proactively include an intentional variety of nutritious foods in your meal plan so that you can ensure that your meals are well-balanced and packed with essential nutrients. Controlling portion sizes is another significant benefit of meal planning, and as we've discussed, how much we eat is a big problem for us Americans. When you set pre-determine serving sizes and prepare meals ahead of time, you create a system that helps you resist the temptation to overeat or set out for unhealthy convenient foods.

When we incorporate educated meal planning and grocery shopping strategies into our lifestyle, we can simplify our healthy eating journey and make it more manageable (and therefore sustainable). Taking the time to plan your meals, shop wisely, and prepare in advance sets the stage for success in achieving your health and nutrition goals. With a well-organized approach and a commitment to making informed choices, you can create a sustainable and enjoyable eating routine that nourishes your body and advances you towards a healthier self.

SELF
SUSTAINED
SHOPPING LIST

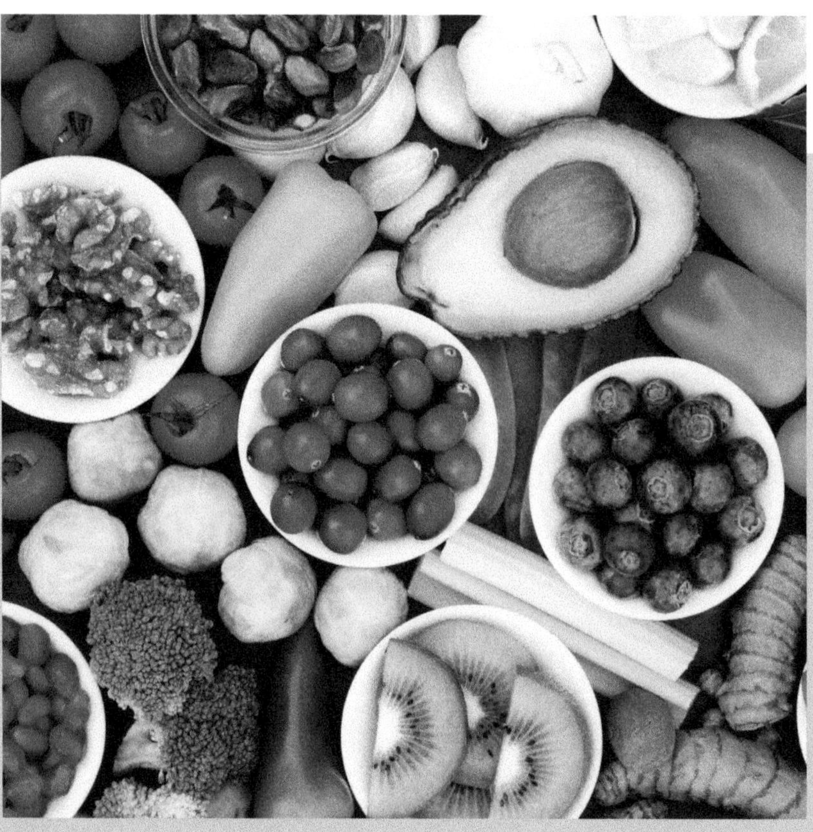

SELF SUSTAINED

12 SUSTAINABLE DIETARY RULES

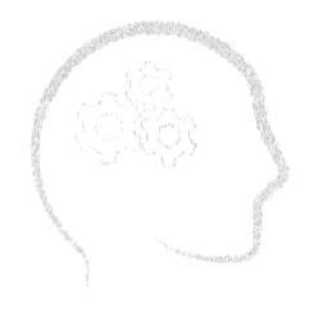

№	DAILY DISCIPLINE CHECKLIST	✓
1	Drink 100 fluid ounces of water	
2	Consume 20-40g Soluble Fiber	
3	Consume less than 40g of sugar; all sugar should be from fruit	
4	***Avoid industrialized SEED OILS .*** *These are under the 'INGREDIENTS' at the bottom of a food label* 1. Soybean Oil 2. Corn Oil 3. Cottonseed Oil 4. Canola Oil 5. Sunflower Oil 6. Safflower Oil 7. Grapeseed Oil For cooking, use **extra-virgin cold pressed olive oil, coconut oil, avocado oil, or beef tallow**	
5	Avoid highly processed foods as much as possible (avoid foods that are packaged with preservatives)	
6	Eat as much ORGANIC food as possible, 70%-100% of diet should be from natural un-processed foods. Your fruits, especially apples and berries, should be organic!	
7	All **beef** should be **organic 100% grass fed** (and preferably *grass finished* as well, but if it says 100% grass fed then it is good enough) All **chicken/turkey meat** should be **organic**, and all **poultry eggs** must be organic ***and pasture raised*** All **fish** should be **wild caught** and not farm raised	
8	Avoid pork for now	
9	Avoid cow dairy/cheeses (especially low quality) (replace with A2 Milk, goat-sheep dairy, macadamia milk, and/or organic + unsweetened almond milk)	
10	Avoid WHOLE GRAINS, legumes (mainly lentils, and peas), corn, and soy. Avoid beans for now, as well.	
11	Avoid uncooked kale and spinach for now	
12	Good nuts and seeds include **walnuts, pecans, pine nuts, macadamia nuts,, hazelnuts, flaxseeds. hemp seeds, sesame seeds, and psyllium seeds.** Avoid cashews, sunflower seeds, pumpkin seeds or peanuts	

Sugar, but more specifically fructose, without fiber tends to cause digestion issues. Soluble fiber is more important than insoluble fiber and is crucial for proper digestion.

These three go together. Most processed foods have industrialized seed oils in them. To avoid this, focus on eating mostly ORGANIC food that is natural and devoid of bad nutrients. Foods that aren't organic are ladened with synthetic pesticides, herbicides, GMO's (genetically modified organisms), and other artificial additives. This will automatically limit foods that are artificial and full of bad nutrients.

80% of commercially raised meat is laced with antibiotics which are BAD. Non-organic animals are also fed industrialized corn/soy/grains, which inflames and damages their body - and we end up eating that tainted meat.

These foods are high in anti-nutrients like lectins. oxalates, and phytates, which are defensive chemicals in plants that disrupts nutrient absorption and destroys our body.

APPROVED FOODS

RESISTANT STARCHES

- ***sweet potatoes***
- ***yams***
- ***yucca***

FLOURS

Gluten-free flours such as:

- ***almond***
- ***coconut***
- ***cassava flour***
- ***rice flour***

NUTS & SEEDS

- ***walnuts***
- ***pecans***
- ***pine nuts***
- ***macadamia nuts***
- ***hazelnuts***
- ***flaxseeds***
- ***hemp seeds***
- ***sesame seeds***
- ***psyllium seeds***

COOKING OILS

- ***avocado***
- ***coconut***
- ***extra virgin olive oil***

MEAT

100% Grass-fed meat (and preferably "grass-finished"), including

- ***beef***
- ***lamb***

Preferably pastured-raised poultry, such as

- ***chicken***
- ***turkey***

("Organic, Non-GMO, No Antibiotic" chicken is good enough)

Wild-caught seafood options, namely:

- ***salmon***
- ***sardines***
- ***shrimp***

DAIRY

Avoid cow dairy/cheeses especially low quality) replace with:

- ***A2 Milk***
- ***goat/sheep dairy,***
- ***macadamia milk***
- ***organic + unsweetened almond milk***

APPROVED FOODS

VEGETABLES

Cruciferous Vegetables:

- ***cabbage***
- ***broccoli***
- ***brussels sprouts***
- ***cauliflower***

Other Vegetables:

- ***asparagus***
- ***beets (raw)***
- ***carrots***
- ***celery***
- ***chicory***
- ***chives***
- ***garlic***
- ***ginger***
- ***horseradish***
- ***mushrooms***
- ***okra***
- ***onions***
- ***parsnips***
- ***radishes***
- ***radicchio***

LEAFY GREENS

- ***Spinach and kale*** should be ***cooked,*** but ***lettuce varieties (red and green leaf lettuces, romaine lettuce)*** can be consumed **raw.**

FRUITS

- ***apples***
- ***apricots***
- ***berries (raspberries strawberries, blackberries, blueberries)***
- ***cherries***
- ***citrus fruits (orange, lemon, lime, etc.) (no juices)***
- ***pears***
- ***kiwis***
- ***nectarines***
- ***peaches***
- ***plums***
- ***pomegranates***

NATURAL SWEETENERS

- ***stevia***
- ***erythritol***
- ***xylitol***

Self Sustained Shopping

APPROVED FOODS

I am least concerned with the list of acceptable foods and more concerned with the foods that you should avoid. Eat in appropriate caloric portions, avoid anti-nutrients, and most foods are fine!

FOODS TO LIMIT OR COMPLETELY AVOID (FOR NOW!)

REFINED, STARCHY FOODS

- wheat flour
- cereal
- cookies
- crackers
- pasta
- pastries
- potato chips
- brown rice
- tortillas

If you're going to eat starchy foods, opt for gluten free options

GRAINS AND GRASSES

- whole grains
- corn
- corn products
- corn syrup
- barley
- brown rice
- kamut
- whole grain oats
- rye
- wheatgrass
- buckwheat
- wild rice

Self Sustained Shopping

FOODS TO LIMIT OR COMPLETELY AVOID (FOR NOW!)

VEGETABLES

- beans* (all, including sprouts and green beans)
- chickpeas* (including as hummus)
- legumes*
- lentils* (all)
- tofu
- edamame
- pea protein
- peas
- soy
- soy protein
- textured vegetable protein (TVP)

FRUITS (SOME CALLED VEGETABLES)

- bell peppers*
- chiles*
- cucumbers*
- eggplant*
- tomatillos*
- tomatoes*
- goji berries
- pumpkin
- squash (any kind)
- zucchini

Any food that is marked with an asterisk (*) must be *deskined/peeled, deseeded, and pressure cooked*. If prepared properly, they do not have to be avoided as much. Beans, for example, if pressure cooked, are a fine staple to a healthy diet.

Self Sustained Shopping

FOODS TO LIMIT OR COMPLETELY AVOID (FOR NOW!)

VEGETABLE OILS

- canola oil (unless it's organic...most are GMO)
- corn oil
- cottonseed oil
- grape-seed oil
- partially hydrogenated oils
- peanut oil
- safflower oil
- soy oil
- sunflower oil
- vegetable oil

MILK PRODUCTS THAT CONTAINS A1 CASEIN

- grain-fed cow dairy; butter, cheese, ice cream, etc.

NUTS & SEEDS

- almonds with peels
- cashews
- peanuts
- pumpkin seeds
- sunflower seeds

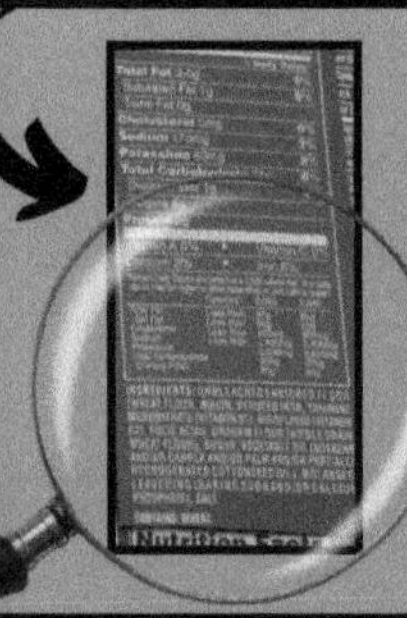

INGREDIENTS: UNBLEACHED ENRICHED FLOUR (WHEAT FLOUR, NIACIN, REDUCED IRON, THIAMINE MONONITRATE (VITAMIN B1), RIBOFLAVIN (VITAMIN B2), FOLIC ACID), GRAHAM FLOUR (WHOLE GRAIN WHEAT FLOUR), SUGAR, VEGETABLE OIL (SOYBEAN AND/OR CANOLA AND/OR PALM AND/OR PARTIALLY HYDROGENATED COTTONSEED OIL), MOLASSES, LEAVENING (BAKING SODA AND/OR CALCIUM PHOSPHATE), SALT.
CONTAINS: WHEAT.

- When examining food labels, your main focus, aside from macronutrients, should be identifying the presence of added seed oils and how many are used. Also check the added sugars! (Reference page 43)

Chapter 10

Embracing Sustainable Eating Habits

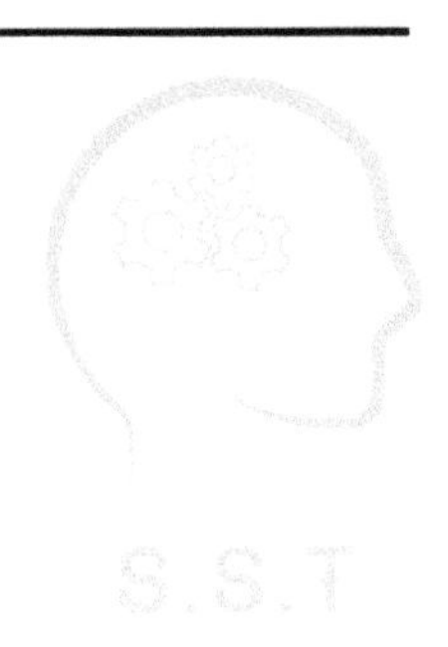

As we reach the end of our remarkable journey together, it's best we reflect on the incredible wealth of knowledge and practical strategies we've uncovered to embrace sustainable eating habits. From demystifying basic nutritional laws to understanding the inner workings of our digestive system, we've developed a competent comprehension of what healthy eating looks like. Now, let's weave together the threads of our exploration and celebrate the empowering potential of adopting sustainable eating habits.

Chapter 1 underscores the inconvenience of pursuing getting healthy. It highlights the conflict between convenience and genuine happiness in the modern world. Convenience offers short-term comfort but doesn't lead to lasting contentment, with the metaphor of water erosion illustrating how small convenient unhealthy choices, like individual droplets within persistent precipitation, accumulate over time to erode our well-being.

It was here where we encouraged you to choose the challenging path of growth and likening it to forging a new trail. It involves sustained effort and swimming against the current of convenience. Chronic inflammation, influenced by dietary choices, and the importance of maintaining gut health are introduced as significant factors affecting our health.

We expressed the importance of a diet rich in anti-inflammatory foods and balancing dietary choices. It concludes by emphasizing *the absence of a one-size-fits-all approach to healthy eating* and encourages small, manageable changes to promote ongoing and worthwhile progress towards a healthier, more fulfilling life.

Then, in Chapter 2, we identified the profound impact of healthy eating on our general health. We explored the fundamental principles of nutrition, diving into the importance of macronutrients, a balanced diet, and portion control. In realizing the role of calories, carbohydrates, proteins, and fats, as well as essential vitamins and minerals, we gained the knowledge to make base-informed decisions about the foods we consume. It was here where we learned about *tracking our food* and looked at *an example of what every meal for a week could look like.* We also explored the concept of energy balance and learning how to maintain a healthy weight through mindful choices and portion control. Knowing about the significance of individual dietary needs and then further exploring different dietary patterns provides us with a comprehensive toolkit for personalized and sustainable eating. Reference Chapter 2 as often as you need!

In Chapter 3, we took a look into the intricate workings of our digestive system. We compared our digestive system to a well-coordinated team of workers in a factory. Just as each worker in the factory has a specific role in the production line, our digestive organs have distinct functions in breaking down food and extracting nutrients. From the moment food enters our mouths to its journey through the esophagus, stomach, small intestine, and large intestine, we witnessed the intricate process of digestion. This newfound knowledge reminds us to slow down, savor our food, chew thoroughly, and be fully present in the nourishing experience of eating. Additionally, we uncovered the pivotal roles of *insulin* and *glucose* in cellular respiration (making energy) and the impact of intermittent fasting on metabolic health.

A central theme emerged in this chapter: the influence of dietary choices on gut health. Chronic inflammation and consumption of inflammatory foods can lead to various disruptions, from serotonin production affecting mood and sleep to over-fermentation in the intestines causing bloated discomfort. Understanding how digestion works empowers us in our quest for healthier living, and knowing about the digestive system sets the stage for the next chapter's exploration on the seductive influence of sugar.

Chapter 4 shed light on the hidden truths about sugar, that sneaky culprit that often creeps into our diets unnoticed. We exposed its detrimental effects on our health, including the risks of obesity, insulin resistance, diabetes, and cardiovascular disease. We explored the different types of sugars, focusing on the detrimental effects of fructose and glucose on hormones and metabolism.

The history of sugar's transformation from being a rare commodity to a processed dietary staple became evident. This shift has had a profound impact on our health, contributing to obesity and various modern diseases, including non-alcoholic fatty liver disease. The importance of reducing sugar intake is emphasized in this chapter, as it affects hunger cues and insulin sensitivity while promoting inflammation. The challenge of identifying hidden sugars in processed foods was addressed, highlighting the need for careful label reading. Practical strategies to cut back on sugar were presented, emphasizing whole, unprocessed foods, mindful beverage choices, home-cooked meals, and gradual sugar reduction. By adhering to recommended sugar limits and fostering awareness, we can take control of our diets, support sustainable healthy living, and relish in the natural sweetness of a balanced diet.

In Chapter 5, we discussed the concept of the fermentability of foods and its effects on gut inflammation. The excessive consumption of alcohol and fermentable sugars, particularly fructose, leads to an overstimulation of the liver and colon, exacerbating inflammation in the gut. Both alcohol and fermentable sugars contribute to liver and gut damage.

The chapter emphasized the importance of distinguishing between fermentable and non-fermentable foods. Fruits and vegetables, rich in soluble fiber, are preferred fermentable foods, supporting healthy digestion. On the contrary, highly fermentable foods like certain grains can worsen gut inflammation. Prioritizing fermentable foods like fruits and vegetables, and avoiding problematic grains, can lead to improved digestion and reduced inflammation. Non-fermentable foods, like lean proteins and non-starchy vegetables, play a vital role in maintaining gut health and effective weight management.

Chapter 5 highlights the need for being mindful of fermentable nutrient intake, especially with alcohol, in the context of individual gut health and tolerance. Alcohol's impact on the body is emphasized, including its prioritization in the liver's metabolic processes and its destructive effect on the gut lining. The chapter exposes the consequences of excessive alcohol consumption, including weight gain, fatigue, and inflammation, which emphasizes the importance of responsible drinking.

In summary, understanding the fermentability of foods is necessary for managing gut inflammation and promoting healthy digestion. Making informed choices about which fermentable and non-fermentable foods to prioritize allows for better control in gut inflammation and optimized nutrient metabolism.

Chapter 6 was all about anti-nutrients; stressing that the quality and quantity of food matters in determining its nutritional impact. The chapter emphasizes that the modern health crisis stems from gluttonous overconsumption, particularly of anti-nutrients found in processed foods.

You were introduced to various anti-nutrients, with a focus on lectins, oxalates, and phytates. We learned how these compounds are present in many plant-based foods, serving as defense mechanisms against predators. When humans consume them in excess, they can pose health challenges. The discussion took this concern and paralleled its dangers to industrialized seed oils and the detrimental effects of their processing methods, which include high-pressure extraction, bleaching, and chemical treatments.

We learned how anti-nutrients resist digestion by human enzymes and can affect the digestive tract's lining, leading to health issues. The extent of these concerns varies among individuals due to everyone having a unique genetic makeup.

Again, this chapter exposes particular anti-nutrients that we should avoid. Lectins, found in grains, legumes, and certain fruits and vegetables, can negatively impact digestive health, especially when consumed raw or undercooked. Traditional methods of cooking, soaking, and fermenting are essential for reducing all anti-nutrient content.

Oxalates, present in leafy greens, vegetables, and fruits, can lead to kidney stones. Cooking and properly preparing oxalate-rich foods can help lower oxalate levels, making them safer for those with sensitivities.

Phytates, prevalent in whole grains, legumes, nuts, and seeds, have antioxidant properties but can interfere with mineral absorption, potentially causing certain nutrient deficiencies.

The chapter raises questions about the trade-offs between the benefits and drawbacks of whole grains and anti-nutrient-rich foods. It is suggested that many of the essential nutrients in these foods can be obtained from other dietary sources, allowing people to minimize their exposure to anti-nutrients. This was then backed by the problematic aspects of industrialized seed oils, which are widely used in processed foods in tandem with highly refined sugar. These oils, when consumed excessively, disrupt the balance between omega-3 fatty acids (anti-inflammatory) and omega-6 fatty acids (pro-inflammatory) - an imbalance in favor of omega-6s, which promotes chronic inflammation. Instead of using canola oil or vegetable oil, substitute them with extra virgin olive oil, coconut oil, or even a high quality butter or ghee. By being aware of certain toxic anti-nutrients, we can begin to make informed dietary choices through a competent understanding how these compounds can affect human health. By doing so, we can begin considering alternatives to harmful anti-nutrients and toxic industrialized seed oils.

In Chapter 7 we harped on practicing mindful eating habits and making smart snacking choices in today's fast-paced world. The combination of these principles will help you develop a healthier relationship with food and promote both nourishment and enjoyment.

Smart snacking is highlighted for its role in providing energy boosts, incorporating essential nutrients, controlling calorie intake, and supporting weight management. We explored various nutritious and satisfying snack options, such as fresh or dried fruits, sliced vegetables, smoothies, and nuts or seeds.

We were also advised to be vigilant about unhealthy snacks and mindless eating, emphasizing the prevalence of processed and refined foods in many grocery stores. The avoidance of seed oils, which are found in numerous packaged and processed foods, is highly recommended. Shopping around the perimeter of the grocery store is suggested to find less processed, healthier options. This is also where we talked about the connection between highly processed foods and mindless eating driven by emotional triggers or boredom. These foods can trigger dopamine release in the brain's reward center, leading to emotional eating patterns and, in some cases, addiction-like behaviors. Recognizing and addressing emotional triggers is crucial for developing a healthier relationship with food.

Planning and preparing wholesome snacks in advance is encouraged to resist the temptation of less healthy choices. This is where we stressed the importance of portion control and mindful eating, which involves savoring each bite, paying attention to sensory experiences, and listening to hunger and fullness cues.

Creating a calm and distraction-free eating environment is recommended, allowing you to focus on the act of eating and show gratitude for nourishment. Planning ahead, mindful portion control, practicing mindfulness, and avoiding distractions contribute to a healthier snacking experience. External influences, such as food marketing and societal pressures, are highlighted as factors that can influence food choices. Remember, you are encouraged to trust yourself and prioritize your own well-being when making food decisions. Ultimately, by integrating mindful eating and smart snacking into daily life, you can develop a healthier and more conscious approach to food. The chapter emphasizes the importance of slowing down, savoring each bite, and choosing nutrient-dense snacks while practicing portion control.

In Chapter 8 we explored the challenges of maintaining a healthy nutrition plan while navigating social situations and dining out. We underlined the importance of social interactions in human life and the need to balance enjoying social experiences with making healthier choices.

The chapter highlights the dual nature of dining out, which offers opportunities to savor delicious food and explore new cuisines but can also present temptations and unhealthy options. Practical strategies and tips were suggested for making healthier choices in such situations.

Planning ahead is a key strategy for dining out. Reviewing the menu online before heading to the restaurant helps identify healthier options and prevents impulsive, less healthy choices influenced by menu descriptions or dining companions. The emphasis is on choosing dishes that incorporate lean proteins and vegetables and avoiding overly-fried foods. Sides and accompaniments are discussed as elements that can significantly impact the nutritional value of a meal. Requesting dietary modifications and replacing high-calorie options like french fries or rolls of bread with healthier alternatives like a salad will enhance the overall dining experience.

Portion control is emphasized due to the tendency for restaurant servings to be larger than necessary. You could always share entrees with dining partners or request take-out containers at the beginning of the meal to avoid overeating.

And speaking of overconsumption, it was this chapter where we touched on the importance of moderation in alcohol consumption during social situations. This was then reiterated by the potential health consequences of excessive drinking. Mixing in glasses of water is suggested to help manage alcohol intake.

Communication with friends and family about your commitment to healthy living is encouraged. Sharing your preferences and dietary goals with them can lead to more accommodating meal planning and foster intimacy and support within relationships. Surrounding yourself with a supportive social network that understands and respects your healthy eating goals is encouraged.

Another alternative to dining out is to gather your social circle and *dine in.* This approach provides more control over food preparation and allows for healthier choices. It's an opportunity to experiment with new recipes and create a more intimate and enjoyable social experience. You can modify this concept by choosing how you hang out with your social circle and choosing activities beyond eating food. Planning activities involving physical movement, activities around town, or anything non-food centered can satisfy social cravings without overindulging in food.

Chapter 9 made meal planning and grocery shopping easy and detailed how to maintain a healthier eating routine. It provides a comprehensive breakdown of the benefits of meal planning, effective strategies for meal planning, and tips for making wise choices during grocery shopping.

We highlighted the time and energy-saving benefits of meal planning. When you plan your meals in advance, you eliminate the need to make daily decisions about what to cook, leading to streamlined cooking processes and reduced stress in the kitchen. Cooking in batches, also known as "meal prepping," is highlighted as a time-saving and convenient approach. Preparing larger quantities of dishes or ingredients ensures readily available meals throughout the week. This approach routinizes the cooking process and promotes consistently efficient ingredient usage. Meal prepping empowers you to make healthier food choices and control portion sizes. By setting predetermined serving sizes and preparing meals in advance, you establish a system that helps resist the temptation to overeat or opt for unhealthy convenience foods.

Meal planning can also lead to financial savings. By creating a well-thought-out shopping list based on your meal plan, you can avoid impulse purchases and minimize wasteful spending. You will also save more money, in the end, by buying higher quality in-store produce and cooking it yourself as opposed to constantly resorting to convenient fast food. This approach encourages you to buy only what you need and fully utilize your ingredients.

Effective meal planning entails dedicating time each week to brainstorm meal ideas, create a menu, and construct a thorough grocery list. This planning process sets the foundation for a successful week of meals and supports positive changes in eating habits. When grocery shopping, having a well-prepared list is crucial. Sticking to this list helps avoid impulse purchases that go against your health goals. The emphasis is on focusing on fresh foods around the store's perimeter, choosing organic and minimally processed options, and reading food labels and ingredient lists attentively.

The emphasis of avoiding seed oils, artificial additives, high fructose corn syrup, artificial sweeteners, food colorings, and artificial flavors is reinforced in this chapter. Instead, we suggest choosing products with natural ingredients, less ingredients overall, and fewer preservatives. High-quality protein sources are recommended, such as grass-fed meats and wild-caught fish.

Incorporating educated meal planning and grocery shopping strategies into your lifestyle simplifies the journey toward healthier eating and makes it more manageable and sustainable. Planning meals, shopping wisely, and preparing in advance set the stage for success in achieving health and nutrition goals. By making well-organized and informed choices, you can create a sustainable and enjoyable eating routine that nurtures your body and builds you toward your healthiest self. Reference the Self Sustained Shopping List as frequent as needed!

Being healthy isn't that hard, and hopefully this book makes getting healthy easier. The essence of "healthy eating" is found in educating your mind and fueling your body appropriately. By threading together the knowledge we've gained in basic nutrition, digestion, sugar management, gut health, anti-nutrients, mindful eating, portion control, social dining dynamics, and the art of smart grocery shopping, we've crafted a sustainable foundation for a lifelong commitment to healthy eating.

We've learned the art of making informed dietary choices and the life changing differences that come with improved eating habits. A cleaner, more nourishing diet doesn't just provide our bodies with essential nutrients; it actively supports the production of beneficial hormones and neural chemicals, including the mood-enhancing serotonin. This dietary transformation not only brightens your mood but also clears your mental fog, granting you newfound mental clarity and emotional stability.

And a more mentally clear and more emotionally stable *you* is capable of much, much more than you currently know. With increased energy, mental clarity, and emotional stability, you'll become a better version of you in all facets of your life. A better *you* is a better friend to your friends, a better partner to your partner, and a better relative to your loved ones.

A better parent to your children.

A better child to your parents.

A better contributing member of society.

A better *you* that will leave a better legacy.

A better human overall.

Remember, embracing healthy eating is a continual journey, and this book serves as your guide to making informed choices and developing sustainable eating habits. As you embark on healthy living, always remember this principle: "*preparation plus opportunity equals luck.*" Each time you actively choose healthier habits over others and choose to live intentionally, you are actively preparing yourself for good luck whenever opportunities in life present themselves. So long you actually prepare to intentionally choose good over bad, healthy over unhealthy, inconvenient over convenient, then you can sleep easy at night knowing you've done enough.

That is integrity. That is accountability.

And integrity and accountability are the keys to unlocking an unwavering faith that allows you to find joy in the journey. Use this book as a reference guide whenever you need to prepare and have no where else to turn to. Even though this book pales in comparison to the genius information that exists out there (especially with the internet, which most of us have nearly 24/7 access to), you can always turn to the pages in this book for guidance and foundational reassurance.

Yesterday is gone, and tomorrow isn't here. Be present today, and you'll see that it's a gift.

Simply **s**tart **t**oday.

Notes

Chapter 1:
[^1] O'Hearn M, Lauren BN, Wong JB, Kim DD, Mozaffarian D. Trends and Disparities in Cardiometabolic Health Among U.S. Adults, 1999-2018. J Am Coll Cardiol. 2022 Jul 12;80(2):138-151. doi: 10.1016/j.jacc.2022.04.046. PMID: 35798448; PMCID: PMC10475326

Chapter 2:
[^1] Sabounchi NS, Rahmandad H, Ammerman A. Best-fitting prediction equations for basal metabolic rate: informing obesity interventions in diverse populations. Int J Obes (Lond). 2013 Oct;37(10):1364-70. doi: 10.1038/ijo.2012.218. Epub 2013 Jan 15. PMID: 23318720; PMCID: PMC4278349

[^2] Lonnie M, Hooker E, Brunstrom JM, Corfe BM, Green MA, Watson AW, Williams EA, Stevenson EJ, Penson S, Johnstone AM. Protein for Life: Review of Optimal Protein Intake, Sustainable Dietary Sources and the Effect on Appetite in Ageing Adults. Nutrients. 2018 Mar 16;10(3):360. doi: 10.3390/nu10030360. PMID: 29547523; PMCID: PMC5872778

[^3] Fernandez ML, Jones JJ, Ackerman D, Barona J, Calle M, Comperatore MV, Kim JE, Andersen C, Leite JO, Volek JS, McIntosh M, Kalynych C, Najm W, Lerman RH. Low HDL cholesterol is associated with increased atherogenic lipoproteins and insulin resistance in women classified with metabolic syndrome. Nutr Res Pract. 2010 Dec;4(6):492-8. doi: 10.4162/nrp.2010.4.6.492. Epub 2010 Dec 28. PMID: 21286407; PMCID: PMC3029790.

[^4] Krebs-Smith SM, Guenther PM, Subar AF, Kirkpatrick SI, Dodd KW. Americans do not meet federal dietary recommendations. J Nutr. 2010 Oct;140(10):1832-8. doi: 10.3945/jn.110.124826. Epub 2010 Aug 11. PMID: 20702750; PMCID: PMC2937576

[^5] The National Academy of Sciences. Dietary References Intakes for Water, Potassium, Sodium, Chloride, and Sulfate. https://www.nap.edu/read/10925/chapter/6#102 Accessed 8/5/2019

Notes

Chapter 3:
[^1] Fish EM, Burns B. Physiology, Small Bowel. [Updated 2022 Oct 14]. In: StatPearls [Internet]. Treasure Island (FL): StatPearls Publishing; 2023 Jan-. Available from: https://www.ncbi.nlm.nih.gov/books/NBK532263/

[^2] Rippe JM, Angelopoulos TJ. Relationship between Added Sugars Consumption and Chronic Disease Risk Factors: Current Understanding. Nutrients. 2016 Nov 4;8(11):697. doi: 10.3390/nu8110697. PMID: 27827899; PMCID: PMC5133084,
Rippe JM, Angelopoulos TJ. Sugars, obesity, and cardiovascular disease: results from recent randomized control trials. Eur J Nutr. 2016 Nov;55(Suppl 2):45-53. doi: 10.1007/s00394-016-1257-2. Epub 2016 Jul 14. PMID: 27418186; PMCID: PMC5174142

[^3] Terry N, Margolis KG. Serotonergic Mechanisms Regulating the GI Tract: Experimental Evidence and Therapeutic Relevance. Handb Exp Pharmacol. 2017;239:319-342. doi: 10.1007/164_2016_103. PMID: 28035530; PMCID: PMC5526216

Chapter 4:
[^1] Temple JL, Cordero P, Li J, Nguyen V, Oben JA. A Guide to Non-Alcoholic Fatty Liver Disease in Childhood and Adolescence. Int J Mol Sci. 2016 Jun 15;17(6):947. doi: 10.3390/ijms17060947. PMID: 27314342; PMCID: PMC4926480.

[^2] White JR Jr. Sugar. Clin Diabetes. 2018 Jan;36(1):74-76. doi: 10.2337/cd17-0084. PMID: 29382983; PMCID: PMC5775006

Chapter 5:
[^1] Guan ZW, Yu EZ, Feng Q. Soluble Dietary Fiber, One of the Most Important Nutrients for the Gut Microbiota. Molecules. 2021 Nov 11;26(22):6802. doi: 10.3390/molecules26226802. PMID: 34833893; PMCID: PMC8624670

[^2] SAMHSA, Center for Behavioral Health Statistics and Quality. 2021 National Survey on Drug Use and Health. Table 2.25A—Alcohol use in lifetime: among people aged 12 or older; by age group and demographic characteristics, numbers in thousands, 2021

Notes

Chapter 6:

[^1] DiNicolantonio JJ, O'Keefe J. The Importance of Maintaining a Low Omega-6/Omega-3 Ratio for Reducing the Risk of Autoimmune Diseases, Asthma, and Allergies. Mo Med. 2021 Sep-Oct;118(5):453-459. PMID: 34658440; PMCID: PMC8504498.

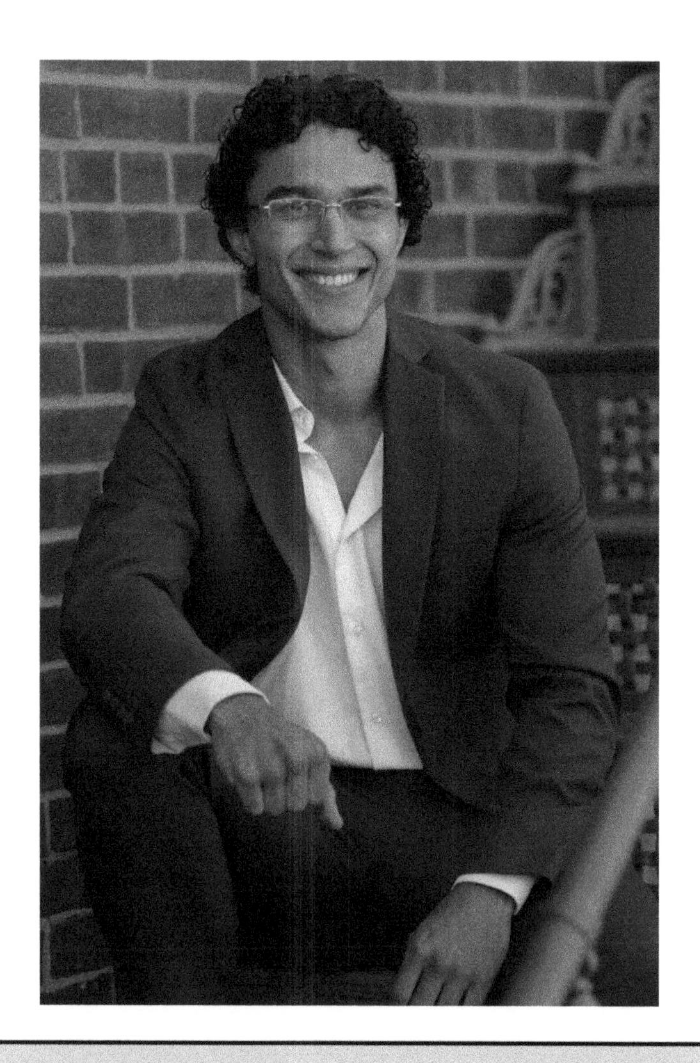

Getting healthy is not hard, it's just inconvenient. If you're willing to pay attention and can learn basic nutrition concepts, you won't need to depend on a health professional ever again. You will become your own health professional. For who knows your body better than you?

About the Author

Mitchell Thompson is a health and wellness professional based out of Kansas City, Missouri. As a seasoned personal trainer and experienced health consultant, he has dedicated his career to helping individuals achieve their health goals and live their best lives.

Mitchell firmly believes that healthy living can be simple and accessible to everyone. This belief has driven him to author this book, *"Healthy Made Easy,"* where he can share his knowledge, expertise, and practical insights to guide readers on their own wellness journey.

With a commitment to making complex health concepts easy to understand, Mitchell combines his years of hands-on experience with a passion for educating and empowering others. In *"Healthy Made Easy,"* he breaks down the fundamentals of nutrition, digestion, and mindful eating, providing readers with the tools to embrace a healthier lifestyle.

Mitchell Thompson is dedicated to creating a positive impact on the lives of readers and helping them achieve their health and wellness aspirations. He hopes that the knowledge and guidance provided in this book will serve as a valuable resource on your path to becoming a healthier, happier you.

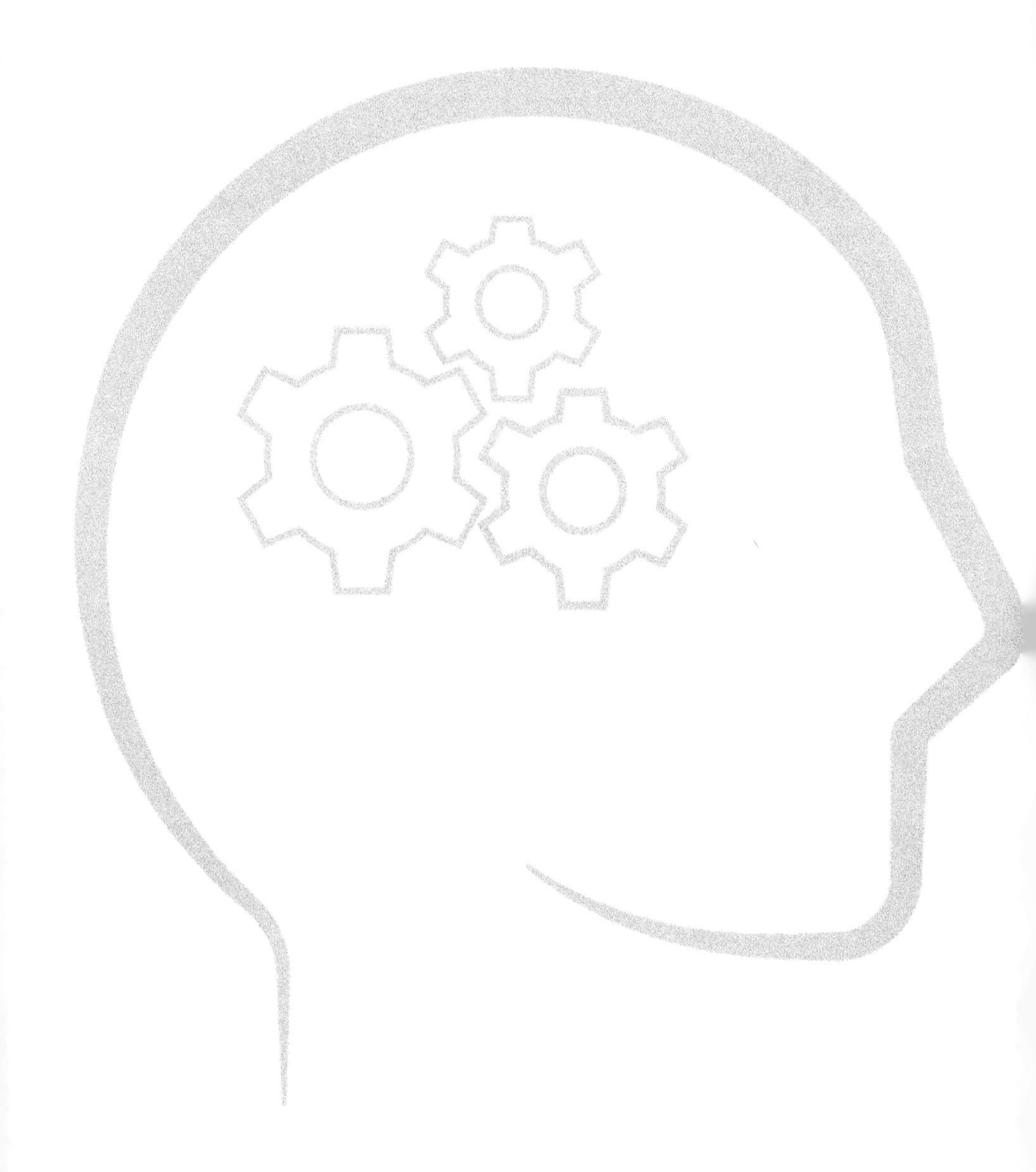

S.S.T